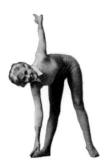

Debbie Drake's
Easy Way To a
Perfect Figure and
Glowing Health

Debbie Drake's
Easy Way To a

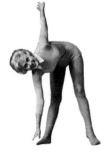

by

Perfect Figure and Glowing Health

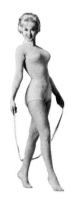

Debbie Drake

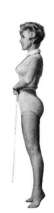

PRENTICE-HALL, INC., ENGLEWOOD CLIFFS, N.J.

EXERCISE PHOTOS BY BURT OWEN

Debbie Drake's Easy Way to a Perfect Figure and Glowing Health,
by Debbie Drake

Library of Congress Catalog Card Number: 61-17883

First printing . . . . December, 1961
Second printing. . . . . . December, 1961
Third printing. . . . . .July, 1962
Fourth printing. . . . . . November, 1962
Fifth printing. . . . . August, 1963

Printed in the United States of America

19704-T

To My Mother
OLA BELLAH
whose patience, encouragement and sacrifice
has made it all possible, and to
LARRY

Acknowledgments

A lot of people have been responsible for making this book a reality. First and foremost is Bob McConnell of the Indiana Broadcasting Corporation, who had the confidence and foresight to give a young girl with an idea the opportunity of really expressing herself through the medium of television. Had it not been for Bob's enthusiasm, planning and hard work many wonderful things would not have happened to me.

Sincere appreciation to Susan Partington, whose help was invaluable in putting my thoughts, and hopes for you, on paper. Ray Reisinger, who has taken great interest in bringing my work to the attention of the public, and Evelyn Konrad, a good friend and wonderful promoter, both of whom deserve a big vote of thanks.

Doctors Art Eberly and Loren Martin have provided me with valuable medical and scientific information on the human body.

There are those who have introduced me to vast audiences—the station managers and owners all over the country and the many sponsors who have shown great faith in my work.

My appreciation also to Dave Smart of WHIO-TV of Dayton, Ohio who believed from the very beginning. To the entire crew at WISH-TV, in Indianapolis, where my program originates, an appreciative thank you for patience and assistance.

To Jim Drinkwater who pioneered with me in this field and taught me so much and to Mrs. Wright, Elizabeth Hale and Toni Frances of Dayton who were with me at the start, another thankful thought.

And last, but not least, to all my wonderful new friends at Prentice-Hall who were so energetic in seeing this book produced, especially John Gudmundsen who edited the material, and Stuart Daniels who has been encouraging, enthusiastic and helpful in many ways.

Table of Contents

Part One

7

Dangers of overweight · How to get rid of that
paunch · Trimmers and toners · Desirable
weights · Reducing diets for men · Hold that
manly pose

A Word
From the Publisher

Never before have Americans been so conscious of their bodies. Good health and a youthful appearance have become part of our national goal. The importance of maintaining a slim, vigorous body as the first step in leading a long, happy life is now generally accepted.

Doctors issue warnings, almost daily, about the dangers of overweight and lack of physical exercise. President Kennedy continually stresses the importance of physical fitness. He has said: ". . . the age of leisure and abundance can destroy vigor and muscle tone as effortlessly as it can gain time. Human activity is rapidly being engineered out of working life. The physical activities that once provided the basis of fitness in youth and later life are rapidly being replaced by machines. And that absence of physical activity is undermining our national physical strength."

The "body beautiful" has become an object not of ego, but of survival.

As the medical and national leaders sounded the alarm, there appeared on the scene, in the last year, a young woman who, through the medium of television, reached into millions of American homes and in a gay and charming way began to teach her viewers ways to improve their health, vigor and personal appearances through easy, interesting daily exercises. The response to Debbie Drake has been overwhelming. By taking exercise out of the realm of drudgery and exhausting gymnastics, and giving it glamour, she has developed an easy, palatable system for achieving physical fitness.

11

Debbie Drake's blonde good looks, scintillating smile and lovely, curvaceous figure are living proof that the system she advocates and demonstrates is truly practical.

As more people became acquainted with Debbie Drake they wanted specific information about their own special problems. They wanted the information in one place for reference. They wanted to be able to do these exercises when business or vacations took them away from their television sets. This book is the answer to the tens of thousands of letters which pour in each month to Debbie Drake.

Debbie Drake, in her meteoric rise to popularity, is more than just another fascinating television personality. She has become a symbol of the physical perfection possible for all who follow her directions. She is her own best example of the benefits to be gained from the guidance to be found within these covers.

What This Book
Will Do for You

This book can be your passport to the beautiful, feminine, youthful figure you would like to have. I can guarantee results because *I know it works.* I learned the hard way. You will be able to learn the easy way, skipping all the mistakes I made.

All of my professional life has been concerned with advising women on the problem of weight reduction and the maintenance of a slim attractive figure. There is little doubt that this matter is a major problem for a large percentage of people in the prosperous, developed areas of the world.

I have discovered a way to achieve the kind of figure most women want. I believe that my system for taking off weight and for developing a slim attractive body is the easiest in the world.

I offer the promise of getting and keeping a glamorous, eye-appealing figure. It is what I call a perfect figure. There is a perfect figure for *you* if you just take a small amount of time to achieve it.

My system isn't hard to follow. In fact it's pleasant to pursue. It has worked for me and for tens of thousands of others. It can work for you. By the time you've finished this book you'll see just what I mean.

Do you know how many minutes there are in every day? One thousand, four hundred and forty (1,440). I ask only that you be willing to give fifteen of those fourteen hundred and forty minutes to having a little fun while you mold your figure to a perfection you never dreamed possible. It isn't a lot to ask of yourself when you consider the results.

What I've Learned

When I was a teen-ager in Dallas, I used to spend my lonely evenings in tears because the boys wouldn't give my scrawny figure even a first look. My dresses never seemed to fit. I became shy and self-conscious. I hated the sight of myself in the mirror. Just as we all do, I longed for a boyfriend who would tell me how nice I looked and who would, with pride, take me to the school dances.

One day I passed a newsstand and my eye was attracted by the lovely girl on the cover of a physical culture magazine. I bought it. That night, covered by the blankets on my bed, I examined the magazine with the aid of a flashlight. I didn't dare let my family know what was in my mind. The next day I did some of the exercises described in the magazine. Day by day I did those exercises behind my bedroom door. Then, I bought more magazines and more books and studied them. My thin body began to fill out and take on more graceful female contours. I began to feel better and found that I could face everyday life with renewed confidence.

Eventually, I enrolled at a local health studio and soon discovered what exercise could really do in shaping the body. But my problems weren't over. I developed a very healthy appetite. Soon, the little, thin, angular girl became a full-blown woman—with many curves—all in the wrong places.

Then I faced the problem so many women face all the time. It's fine to have curves, but what do you do when you have too many of them and they are really more like bulges? So I learned the second part of the secret of keeping a beautiful, perfect figure! Namely, that good, sound common sense is needed when the dinner bell rings.

I've learned a lot more since then. And, I'm eager to tell you all about it. In this book you'll find many ideas which will help you to lead a happy, well-balanced life. You need never be hungry while reaching for your ideal weight. You need never be tired as you achieve your perfect figure. As a matter of fact you'll feel more energetic than ever before as you give up

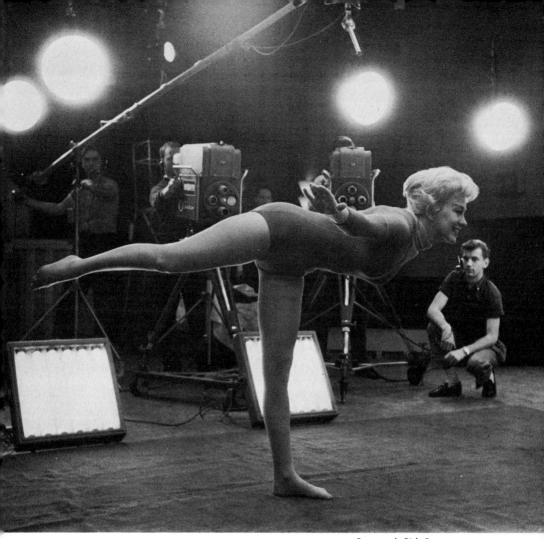

Ben and Sid Ross

I usually get my fifteen minutes of daily exercise in front of the TV cameras. My system for gaining and keeping a slim, attractive figure is the easiest in the world to follow, I believe. Here I'm demonstrating an exercise to keep the midriff slim, at WISH-TV in Indianapolis.

unwanted pounds and feel your body become firm and supple.

All of this I learned the hard way. I hope you'll follow the easy path I've charted in these pages. Since those days in Dallas, I've devoted myself to helping men and women achieve the figures and weights nature intended them to have. I have studied and I have taught. A few years ago I managed a group of health and reducing salons which operated in many cities all over the United States. More recently, on television, first in

15

Indianapolis and then in dozens of other cities, I've had the privilege of instructing and demonstrating to millions of people how really healthy they can become and how easy it is for women to achieve their own perfect figure. To those of you who regularly follow me on the air I've given a great deal of information for which you've asked. For the others, I hope this book opens up a whole new wonderful world.

Debbie Drake

P.S. Although this book is primarily for women, there is a great deal in it for every man. There is even a section "For Men Only" but the girls may read it, if they wish. In fact, I hope they will do so and then recommend this book to their favorite males. Too many men are being lost every day to heart attacks and other ailments that are caused by, or are traceable to, overweight. We women don't like to see our men leave this life before their time. So, I'll continue to do my best to help keep them with us.

D.D.

Part One

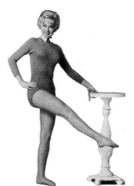

Your
Passport
To Figure Beauty
And Vital Health

1

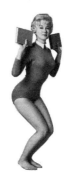

You and Your Figure

Are you ready to start down the road to health and happiness AND *the* perfect figure? What are we waiting for—let's get going and start trimming away that excess poundage.

First of all, as a professor would say, let's define our terms. Just what do we mean by *"the* perfect figure?" Very simply this: the perfect figure is that figure which is in proper proportion with regard to bone structure, weight, height and frame. The perfect figure varies from person to person. Audrey Hepburn has an excellent figure, yet her measurements are quite different from Sandra Dee's, and both actresses are nearly the same height. Audrey Hepburn has a gamin, elfish quality, while Sandra Dee reminds us of what she is: an exuberant, bubbling teen-ager—pert and pretty. What about Marlene Dietrich who bounces grandchildren on those famous legs? She is beyond the so-called prime of woman's life, yet her figure is lovely and graceful. You can find people in every walk of life—actresses, women in the fashion and advertising fields, as well as wives and mothers who know the important ingredients of exercise and proper eating habits in healthy happy lives.

Age Isn't the Problem

These days it's often hard to tell a mother from her daughter. I have a friend who is a department manager in the Junior Size shop of a well-known store. She told me the other day that she often sees two girls come into the department—both dressed in Bermuda shorts, both wearing sneakers and white oxford, button-down blouses. Both of them have scrubbed,

17

shiny faces and clear, alert eyes. It's only when one of the girls says, "How do you like this dress, Mother?" that it's obvious that they are mother and daughter, and not two girl friends on a shopping spree.

A Good Figure Is a Health Asset

It isn't only the desire for a perfect figure that leads women to watch what they eat and to exercise. Doctors, insurance companies and statistics bear out one grim fact: excess weight is not an asset; it is a definite liability. Your doctor will tell you that when a woman is at her ideal weight, she greatly reduces those odds and ends of aches and pains that constantly plague her. Not only that, but there is a big increase in morale and self-confidence, and even a livelier step as she walks down the avenue.

So, we can pretty definitely state that the perfect figure is not the figure of the girl who wins the Miss America Contest or the Miss Rheingold Contest or that of Sophia Loren or Angie Dickinson. These girls all have perfect figures. But they don't have *your* perfect figure. You don't have to look like them, or any other public personality or motion picture star, to have a perfect figure.

Nor is the perfect figure limited to that of a young girl of eighteen or twenty. Figure perfection can easily be kept into the forties and fifties and even beyond. Remember, it is not dependent on any one factor—height, body structure or age. It is the figure which is perfect for YOU—not the girl next door or up on the movie screen.

Understand Your Body Type

Your ideal or perfect figure is achieved when you understand your general body type and make the very best of what you have. Don't ever say "I'll never have the figure of a chorus girl or model, so I don't care." This attitude causes you to overeat and let your waist thicken with unwanted fat. Remember, you can be perfect for *your* size and physical structure.

Look around at the girls you see in the office, the super-market, at the beach or walking along the street. How many of them would have lovely figures if they held themselves a little straighter, or took two inches off their waists and added them to their bustlines? These things I guarantee you will be able to do while reading and using this book.

Some of the loveliest girls I know, whose figures draw many an eye, wouldn't meet the model specifications of 34–24–34. I'm thinking of one girl whose hips are a little too broad to meet the so-called ideal figures because her hip bones are made that way. Yet, by keeping her weight down and doing the proper exercises to assure herself a slim waistline, she presents one of the loveliest appearances of anyone I've ever seen. Most of us have some physical drawback—ankles thicker than they should be, too large a rib cage, a tendency to gather fat around the thighs, or any number of other figure faults. The great majority of these can be corrected. Some of these drawbacks, because they are based on basic bone structure which cannot be altered, can still be minimized. But, and this may be the most important thing you'll learn from this book, you can do something *really spectacular* in correcting most of your figure faults.

Be Yourself

Remember! Don't try to look like someone else. Be yourself but be your best self. I'll do my best to help you discover charms you never dreamed you had.

As our ideas and times change, so do our visual tastes. Venus de Milo could stand in the town square for days before she'd get a wolf whistle from today's young gentlemen. And Renoir's bathing beauties might hang over a sofa in a bachelor's apart-ment, but you can be sure that the gal he's curled up with on that sofa is probably a size Nine or Ten. She might even be a Seven or Eight, if he's lucky. Men may decry the hollow-cheeked faces that peer from fashion magazines, but the girl with Santa Claus cheeks will be put into the "best buddy" class . . . not the "best girl" class.

But back to the perfect figure and you. I guess now you can see how important it is, not only for the sake of appearance, but more important for the sake of health.

Your Ideal Weight

Next term: what is the ideal weight for your height? The weight charts in this book are modern. Old weight charts based on the national averages are as outdated as the hats we once wore. We have since found out that the typical American is about ten pounds overweight. It has recently been discovered that your most desirable or ideal weight is ten pounds less than average. Remember that this is a medical conclusion based on statistics which show that you can live longer and have fewer illnesses when you are slender. But achieving the proper number on the scales isn't the only thing that makes the perfect figure—there's another little fact that plays a big part: how those pounds are distributed. Is yours an hourglass figure with all the sand at the bottom and time running out at the top? Or has time stood still at high noon? That's where exercise comes into its own.

It is generally accepted that the most attractive shaping of the female form is this: a firm, high, rounded bustline, a narrow waist, gently curving hips, tapering legs and slender arms. And the men who watch for figures like this don't care how they are clad: whether in toga or tights, bustle or bikini.

As with every ideal there are variations on the theme. Think of how many adjectives you could give to the various kinds of perfect figures and then associate them with people in the public eye. Stately—Ingrid Bergman; willowy—Marlene Dietrich; petite—Lily Pons; voluptuous—Marilyn Monroe; cuddly—Sandra Dee. All different, yet all perfect in their own ways. So should you be.

The perfect figures of some actresses, models, career girls, wives, mothers aren't accidents. If you hear the remark that Sally, or Diana, or Marjorie, has a perfect figure because she is lucky, remember this definition of luck given by one far wiser than I—*Luck:* good planning, carefully executed. The perfect figure is the result of proper eating, a daily program of light exercise and the will to have a perfect figure. That is the kind of luck that is involved.

Know Yourself

It's as important today as when Socrates said it more than two thousand years ago: "Know thyself." Shakespeare also said it, perhaps a little more poetically. "To thine own self be true."

Let's start being true or honest with ourselves. Have you ever studied your figure? I mean really studied it? Not just looked in the mirror briefly while hooking a bra or fastening a stocking to utter a heart-rending "Ugh."

All work and no play can make a dull girl, indeed. Hobbies are excellent for your spirits. I'm taking flying lessons from world-famous aviator Roscoe Turner, who is shown here welcoming me aboard a plane at the airport near my home in Indianapolis.

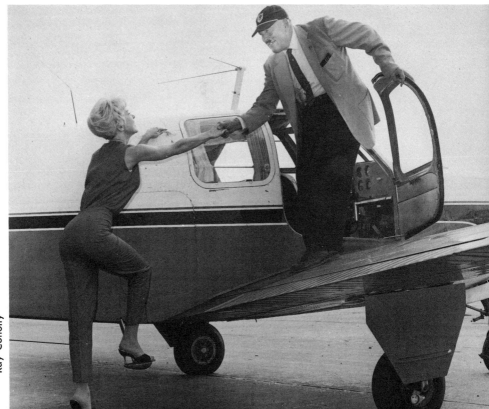

Ray Conolly

Most women are used to seeing themselves in some form of clothing—usually with a tight foundation garment underneath to improve the picture. They have long forgotten what their own bodies actually look like.

Start right now by taking a good look at yourself. Strip right down to your birthday suit and examine yourself in a mirror . . . front, back and profile. Girdles and brassieres may fool the world into believing your figure is fine—but you shouldn't make the mistake of letting these props fool you, too.

Take a good long look at yourself and then remind yourself that you can improve any part of your figure that needs it. There is an exercise for every type of figure fault.

Pinch a bit here and there to analyze your body for firmness and overweight. Can you pick up layers of loose skin between your fingers?

Carefully examine every part of your body and note on a piece of paper when you see areas which need improvement.

Neckline and Chin:	Any extra fat here? Check for loose folds of skin. This is a telltale area for giving away your age.
Shoulders:	Slumped or drooping shoulders are posture faults that destroy the beauty of the upper torso. Give yourself a posture check (page 33).
Back:	Plump little folds of fat often sneak in across the back.
Bust:	Too large or too small? Firm or droopy?
Waist:	Is it as slim as it might be? Can you hold more than two inches of flesh between your fingers?
Hips:	Too much padding? Or not enough curves?
Buttocks:	Round and firm—or has the sag hit here, too?
Thighs:	The bathing suit season reminds us all of the importance of keeping the thighs

	slim and firm. Are there extra pads of fat on your thighs? Or are they too straight and undeveloped?
Calves:	Shorter skirts make us more leg-conscious. Heavy calves can be trimmed down; skinny legs built up.
Ankles:	Even thick ankles can be slimmed down by exercise. Or is your problem that they are not full enough?
Feet:	These poor things bear the brunt of carrying overweight and being crowded into tight shoes.

Are you happy with what you saw in the mirror? The chances are you aren't. However, there is no need to despair. You are going to be able to have the figure you want—your perfect figure—no matter how impossible it may seem to you right now.

It might be interesting to find out how we develop the kinds of figures we have. Your figure is a direct result of your daily habits. No one was born to be fat. Fatness, obesity or overweight, whatever you want to call it, is not inherited. The tendency toward it, along with height and frame, are the factors involved. Bad eating habits are inherited in that they are passed down from mother to daughter, generation to generation. Overweight is caused by one thing: excess food. If this is combined with a lack of physical activity that allows the body to go soft and flabby, what can you expect but a dumpy upside-down figure? The natural design of the female form is one of beauty and grace. You can keep it that way with just a little time and effort.

Glandular Deficiencies

In some cases, overweight is caused by improper balance of the glandular functions. However, with rare exceptions, this problem need not prevent a woman from improving her figure.

A doctor can help right nature's wrong. Modern medicine has found the means to restore the natural balance and regulate the absorption of food.

If you find it impossible to lose weight or have a tendency to gain no matter how little you eat, then it is wise to consult your physician. He will be able to determine the kind of medication and treatment you may need if your problem is caused by some glandular malfunction. On the other hand, the problem of extreme thinness and inability to gain weight is often due to overactivity of a specific gland. A visit to your physician may also help you to correct this condition.

2

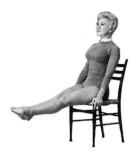

Just Fifteen Minutes
a Day

The secret of the perfect figure lies in regular daily exercise, not fifteen minutes today and fifteen minutes next week. That's one thing I want you to promise me and yourself—that you will spend fifteen minutes every day doing the exercises—with no excuses. It's only by exercising fifteen minutes every single day including Saturdays and Sundays that your muscles will begin to take on tone, the bulges disappear and your new figure begin to emerge.

The exercises you include in your fifteen-minutes-a-day depend upon the figure problems you are trying to solve. In the second part of this book I describe exercises for every area of the body. But I want you all to start off with the Basic Six which you'll find starting on page 109.

Nature works for you in many strange and wonderful ways. One of her little miracles is called the natural girdle. The girdle you buy is mostly made of elastic material. As you wear and wash this garment, much of the elasticity disappears and pretty soon you have to get another one. Nature puts out a girdle, guaranteed not to wear out—and, as a matter of fact, the more you use this natural girdle the stronger it becomes. This natural girdle is made up of your muscles. These muscles slim, tighten and control the contours. The more they are pulled and stretched, the more resilient they become. It is only when the muscles are not used that they become soft and flabby and lazy. When muscles are not kept busy, any unusual exertion brings aches and pains.

The particular part of us which seems to resist this natural girdle is the tummy. Even though overeating causes a more general gain of weight, you may nevertheless feel that your tummy has become more obvious, so you invest in a good tight girdle. You may feel you look slimmer, but chances are you are less comfortable than you would be if you could rely on your stomach muscles to do the job for you as nature intended. I am certain you will agree that it is much more desirable and much less expensive not to have to depend on this artificial means. If you will take just fifteen minutes a day to follow my program, you can teach these muscles to do the task naturally.

Your First Exercise

Right now, I assume you're sitting in a comfortable chair reading this. Start to work on your first exercise. You can easily flex the muscles in the stomach at will. If you consciously pull these muscles in over and over again you will soon have them so well trained that you won't have to command them. The muscles will work by themselves. The muscles of the upper arms are another example of what happens when natural flexing movements are seldom employed. You'll never see flabby arms on an active child. He's too busy climbing trees or running or playing ball. A full-grown woman hasn't the desire to run or climb trees. As a result of no activity for the arm muscles, the flesh begins to sag and the muscles get lazy. But there are exercises that can give women the same result as if she had skipped rope or climbed a tree. You'll see what they are when we get to the section which describes the exercises.

Again, let me repeat: age is no factor. Look at Gloria Swanson. Here is a wonderful example of what exercise can do for a woman. Miss Swanson proudly admits her age. Yet her body is slender and firm.

Miracles Can Happen

One of the most miraculous examples of what exercise can do to re-shape the body happened when I worked with a woman in Columbus, Ohio. She was in her late forties and weighed 255 pounds. Her skin hung in loose folds over her body. Huge layers of fat drooped from her thighs. The fat on her back lay in pleats. I put her on a reducing diet and outlined a program of exercise to accompany it. The weight loss came gradually but easily. I questioned, however, the possibilities of ever restoring the huge, flabby body to firm proportions—particularly as every pound that disappeared would leave more stretched skin behind. She exercised faithfully along with her diet. In six months she had lost 60 pounds. She was still highly overweight at 195 pounds—but the change in her appearance is almost impossible to describe. Miraculously, this woman who had for so long been a towering mountain of flesh—acquired a shape! The folds disappeared. Though she was still heavy, she now had the proportions of a woman. Her bustline was full and attractive. Her back became firm. There was a definite indentation at the waist, a gentle curve to the hips. Her thighs firmed. Most surprising was the tummy. It flattened out beautifully; became firm and tight. She was so thrilled with these results that she wrote me a letter of appreciation which I will always cherish. One of the unforgettable expressions she used was that she had gained a feeling of completeness about her body which was a new experience. She said that her body had always seemed to move in sections. Now she felt pulled together and in control of her body movements. She was determined to continue her program until she could wear a size 14 dress and at last report—she was nearing her goal. It happened to her and she really had a problem—it can happen to you. Let me repeat: diet took off the excess pounds for this woman, but it was exercise that gave her a figure.

Start Slowly and Work Up Gradually

Think of yourself as a sleepy bear just emerging from its winter hibernation. You and your muscles have been asleep for a long time. First a little yawning and stretching—then some waking-up exercises, and before you know it you'll have a set of muscles that are wide awake, alert and alive. They may resist at first, but keep at it. They'll begin to enjoy the exercises. It's just that exercises are something new to these muscles.

Here's something to be careful about: don't overdo the exercising at the beginning. Work up to a varied and longer program slowly. Though you may feel like doing twenty-five or fifty repetitions of an exercise in the beginning, do only five the first day. Work up to twenty-five slowly over a period of one or two weeks.

When and Where to Exercise

Any time is the right time for exercise. It may be morning, noon or night. Some women get up fifteen minutes earlier each morning and do their exercises before anyone else is awake. In some families everyone does the exercises together. If it suits your schedule better to exercise in the evenings, by all means do so, although you may be less inclined to do so. If time is really a problem split the fifteen minutes into five-minute sessions scattered throughout the day. Just be careful to wait a half hour after a light meal and a full hour after a large meal before exercising.

You have just as much freedom in choosing where to exercise as when. The living room usually offers more open floor space but it can also be the bedroom or playroom. Choose any place that gives you enough room to spread your arms wide, to do full kicks forward and backward without taking that precious vase off the table, and with enough floor space so that you can stretch out full length.

None of my exercises calls for professional equipment. Everything you need can be found in your own home. One of my students uses an old mattress pad for lying on the floor. Two straight chairs, a few pillows and the edge of your bed or couch are all that are necessary. Books or canned goods make ideal weights for the gaining exercises. And your ironing board is easily converted into a slant board. The important factor is your determination. You could have the best equipment in the world, but it won't do a thing for you unless you do these exercises regularly. One of my TV students wrote me recently that she followed my program faithfully but that she was unable to do some of the high kicks and wide arm reaches because she lived in a trailer and there wasn't enough room. Here's a girl with the right amount of determination. She wants her new figure and she'll get it come what may.

Another TV viewer is a farmer's wife with eight children, ranging from two to thirteen. The whole family does the exercises with her. As she puts it, when the Debbie Drake program is on the air, you can't get through the living room.

What to Wear

I wear a leotard on my TV show because it is comfortable and enables the viewer to follow my movements. For early morning exercises you may wish to stay in pajamas or nightgown. Shorts or slacks are ideal. The important thing in choosing an exercise outfit is that you have complete freedom of movement for your arms and legs, and that nothing is tight or binding, especially at the waist.

How Soon Can You Expect Results?

Every woman I work with always asks the same question. "How long will it take before I see results?" I can't give you a definite answer. It depends upon how much change is required and upon how your system reacts to the new diet and exercise.

The waistline will be the first place to see results. As a general rule, the larger you are, the quicker you will lose inches. If you stick to your daily routine of diet and exercise, with as many as thirty repetitions of three or four waist exercises, you could expect to lose as much as 3½ inches the first month. It is often harder to go from a 26-inch waist to a 24-inch waist than to decrease one from 35 inches to 30 inches. Hips can be reduced 2 to 4 inches a month by a large person. The thighs take longer to reduce and firm than any other area. One to two inches a month is a very good loss to look for in the thighs.

Increasing, particularly in the bustline, is a slower process than losing inches. We can add on to the waist and stomach easily enough by overeating, but building up in other areas is more difficult. Do not be discouraged if you show no significant changes for as long as two months. The increase *will* come.

One of my students in Dallas—a woman in her thirties—had had a small bust and large hips since her teens. Her hips measured 42 inches and her bust 32 inches. With my diet and exercise plan, her bust increased from 32 inches to 34 inches and the hips went down to 38 inches in just three months. She went on to improve these measurements to a 35-inch bust and 37-inch hips which to her had seemed an impossible ideal.

I had a student in Birmingham who contradicted all the general rules about building up. This girl had been painfully thin all her life. Whenever she did manage to add a few pounds, they went directly to her abdomen. We worked together on a gaining diet and exercise program and in two months she had added 4 inches to her bust, 2 inches to her hips, 1½ inches to her thighs, yet she managed to keep the tiny waist she had always had. It has happened to others. It can happen to you. The important thing is to set your goal and stick to it. You will find yourself looking forward eagerly to your exercise routines. Each week you will see and feel the improvements in your appearance, your body tone and your general vitality.

You know how good a drink of cool water is. Think how good a lungful of fresh air is for your body. Fresh air and deep breathing at an open window give your complexion and body a lift. Make sure your exercise room is well-ventilated.

It is a good idea, as well as a refreshing one, to follow your exercise period with a bath or shower. This will assure personal daintiness and wash away any perspiration. A cool rinse afterwards is just the perfect set-me-up for the day. If you exercise in the evening, soak in a warm tub to relax you and prepare you for a good night's sleep.

Think Your Way to a Perfect Figure

Every move you make with your body is an exercise. To exercise the body means merely to use it. But you can exercise to a goal just as easily as you can exercise toward overweight.

Breathing exercises the lungs; walking, the legs; reading, the eyes; and thinking, the brain. Once you get into the habit of "thinking" exercise, you can turn almost any ordinary movement into an aid to your perfect figure. The exercises which follow can be done in the course of your daily rounds. They should *supplement* your basic program of fifteen minutes a day and not be regarded as a substitute.

Chair-rising: How many times a day do you get up from a chair? Dozens! Up from the breakfast table, up from an office desk, up from your living room chair—over and over again through the day you are rising from a chair without thinking about it. Yet here is a chance to do one of the most effective exercises for the hips and thighs I know.

Instead of getting up in your usual way, keep the feet close together in front of the chair and rise slowly without using your hands for support. Keep your back straight as you come up. You will feel the pull through the thighs. If you sit down again in the same manner, back straight and no hand support—you will double the benefits.

Leg-holding: There is another easy exercise that requires no special time or effort. It is an excellent firmer for the thighs.

While sitting on a straight chair, raise one leg off the floor and hold it straight out in front of you. Be sure you lift the knee and thigh slightly off the chair seat. Hold the leg in a suspended position for as long as you can. Release and alternate with the other leg. Do this often while you are watching television. It is so easy, so effective. If you can hold both legs up at the same time, you will get double value, for it increases the pull.

Reaching: Any strong pull from the arms to the waist will slim and limber the upper torso. Right now, you are probably doing many arm reaches through the day. If you play my "Think Exercise" game, you can make each of these movements a reach toward beauty.

When putting the glassware and china away, do it piece by piece, rather than in groups and stacks. I make a point of putting the things I use most on higher shelves. This may horrify the efficiency experts but it gives me a chance for extra beauty reaches every day.

You can get the same beauty benefits when putting books back on the shelves. Put them up one by one. Make each reach a strong stretch. This will firm and lift the bosom. It will keep the upper arms tight and youthful, too.

Bending: Every time you bend down to pick up the children's toys, you can slim your waistline and tighten your tummy. Stand with your feet slightly apart and bend over from the waist. Pick them up one by one. Up come the toys— off go the inches.

Stair-climbing: Do you usually take the elevator to your office floor? Do you live in an apartment building with elevator service? You have a wonderful chance to trim down your hips and slim your thighs. All you have to do is walk up a few flights, instead of riding, once a day. Lift the knees high at each step to get the maximum pull on the muscles.

Toe-walking: The minute I get inside my front door, off come my shoes and I walk around my house on my toes. This is wonderful for the arches and it slims the ankles and calves. It is also a great tonic for tired feet.

Going up and down on your toes as often as possible is a fine exercise for the legs. While waiting for the kettle to boil, the soup to simmer—or any other spare moment—raise and lower yourself up and down on your toes. Once you start *thinking* about it, you will find many chances to do this throughout the day.

Tummy-pulling: One of the best exercises for the abdominal muscles is simply to pull them in. Take deep breaths and pull in as hard as you can. Let the breath go, but keep the tummy in. There are so many chances to do this in a day, I can't count them. To develop the habit, start with special reminders. Every time you wait in line at the grocery store, for instance, could be your signal to practice tummy holding. If you do a lot of walking (and I hope you do), make it a habit to pull in the tummy as you wait for the traffic light to change. These plans will help you get started. Soon you will be doing it automatically and you are on your way to a nice flat tummy forever.

Chin-lifting: Tilt your head back and lift your chin as high as you can. Move the chin up and down with strong pulls, strong enough for you to feel them through the neckline. This may look a little strange to anyone catching you at it—but it is a wonderful way to keep a youthful throat line. Beauty is as beauty thinks—and when you remind yourself about figure improvement, you can automatically *do* something about it.

Finger-flexing: Youthful, graceful hands are a part of your perfect figure. You can improve the flexibility and even the shape of your hands whenever you think about them. Whenever your hands are free, stretch out the fingers. Pull them as widely apart as you can. Make tight fists—then open them quickly and flex the fingers. Shake the hands often. It will send the blood tingling through them and improve the circulation. No need to devote time from your fifteen-minutes-a-day to hand exercises. You can work these in often without taking any special time for them.

Posture Practice: John Robert Powers, the model expert, taught me this trick for posture improvement. When you ride in an elevator, try to move into a position against the elevator wall. Line your body up against the wall. The head, the shoulders, the waist and the buttocks should be pushed against the wall. Pull yourself up to full height. Your body will now be in perfect posture alignment. Maintain this model pose as you leave the elevator.

Eye-rolling: These precious members of the body deserve some special treatment, too. Exercise your eyes by rolling them. Look as far off to the right as you can—then up—then off to the left, then down. Keep your head straight as you do this. It is the eyes we are exercising this time, not the neck. If you are "thinking" exercise, you will find many convenient times to practice this.

Hair-brushing: You can make hair brushing a figure exercise. Hold the brush firmly, and with strong arm movements brush through the hair. Let the wrists flex with each stroke. You will be lifting the bust, firming the arms and adding grace to your gestures—while you put a sheen in your hair.

If you can do your hair-brushing while lying down, so much the better. Let the head drop off the end of the bed or sofa. You will increase the circulation, which will improve the complexion and stimulate the hair growth. If you lie on your back with your head tilted backwards, you will firm the neck muscles as you brush.

Had you ever thought about how many other beauty benefits could be derived from the simple routine of brushing your hair?

Face-cleansing: This is another beauty ritual which you probably follow twice a day. To get extra value out of it, be sure you apply your cleansing cream with firm, upward strokes. Give the chin and neck special attention—gently pushing the skin upward. This way you will not only cleanse your skin but give the facial muscles a toner, too. Upward movements keep the face and throat firm and youthful.

Body-lotioning: I am very fond of body lotions and always use a generous amount of them after my bath or shower. When applying lotion, give yourself a body massage. Always work with upward motions. The direction of youth is up: all downward lines are aging lines. Push firmly with both hands up from the ankles and around the calves. Knead the lotion into the thighs. Do the same with the arms, starting from the hands and wrists and working upward. Work the lotion in well around the tummy, pressing in on these muscles. Massage the breasts: lift them up and work with circular finger motions.

How to Select Your Exercises

Every woman, whether she is young or old—fat or thin—or just right . . . should do one exercise every day for her bust, waist, hips and thighs, upper arms and neckline. These are the beauty basics. They will assure you of a trim, youthful firm figure throughout your lifetime. You can double the Basic Six to a daily dozen by adding an additional exercise for each of these areas. These are the beauty duets. By doing two different exercises for each part of the body, you increase the values of each. One works in partnership with the other. You will get better results this way than you would by doing the same exercise twice as many times.

Start with five to seven repetitions of the Basic Six exercises for the first three days. After the third day, add one repetition for each until you reach 10 for gaining, 25 or more for reducing. At the beginning of the second week, you are ready to add more exercises to your routine. Work up to three or four exercises for each problem area. For reducing, do as many counts as possible for each exercise—up to 45, if you can. For gaining, you should exercise with weights only every other day.

If you are one of the lucky girls whose weight is correct and whose measurements are well-proportioned, you should continue the Basic Six exercises and add two or three additional exercises for each of these areas, doing as many repetitions as possible in the fifteen-minute period. This will keep you in all-around perfect condition. I like a lot of variety in my own exercise routine and change my selection of basics regularly. If your weight and measurements are correct, chances are your muscle tone is better than average. You should be able to work into a full fifteen-minute program within a week's time.

If you have extreme figure problems, you may want to devote more time to your exercise program than just fifteen minutes. That is up to you. If you get to be as enthusiastic about exercising as I am, you may very well want to do more.

Your Figure and Your Posture

It's an old rule, but a true one—any figure, fat, thin, flat or full, is more attractive when it is carried well. Fat women look so much better when they stand tall. Skinny girls make the most of their limited curves by holding their shoulders back and their chests out. Older women look years younger with youthful, buoyant movements that come with better posture. And teen-agers gain needed poise when their posture is graceful.

It's easy to have good posture. As with exercise, you must *think* good posture. Hold your head high, not tilted as if you were studying the clouds, but high, like a proud-stepping stallion. Pretend that you are trying to push the top of your head through the ceiling. But keep your chin parallel to the floor. Relax your shoulders. Don't strain them either forward or backward. Lift the chest and bustline by stretching upward through the midriff and pulling up at the back of the neck.

Pull in your stomach and abdomen by contracting the abdominal muscles. This will make your bosom lift as well.

This is important whether you are sitting or standing. You can practice while you are at your desk, sitting at the dinner table, riding a bus, wherever you are seated.

When you are standing, remember to tuck your hips under. The lower spine should be relaxed. Any hard pull on the lower back will eventually result in a sway-back which no one wants or needs. The knees, which are the shock absorbers of the body, should be kept relaxed also. If you have trouble keeping your shoulders back, or have round shoulders, try this trick. Bend your elbows and try to touch them together behind your back. This will help straighten the shoulders and will relieve tensions in the upper back.

A New Slant on Beauty

One of the problems in beauty and health is the circulation of blood. Every moment we stand, sit or walk the blood is being pulled downward. When we reverse the position, letting the blood flow freely into all the corners it ordinarily misses, it refreshes the skin and improves the circulation. The easiest way to effect this is to raise the feet higher than the head.

The Yogis stand on their heads for prolonged periods of time. Indra Devi, one of the leading exponents of Yoga in this country, describes the benefits of headstanding in her book *Yoga for Americans.* Lady Mendl, the world-famous decorator, was an international beauty in the 'nineties. Her secret: she stood on her head for a few minutes every day throughout her life. Billy Burke starts every day with a headstand.

If headstanding is a little too rigorous for your taste, you can reap the same reward from a slant board. I use an ordinary ironing board. It is comfortably padded and just the right length. Put the narrow end against a chair, seat or sofa. Lie down with the feet stretched upward and the head down. Five to fifteen minutes in this position will put sparkle in your eyes, relieve tension and give your skin fresh radiance. Here's another secret: if you have to go out in the evening after a busy day and you don't have time for a nap, set your hair, put cold cream on your face, eye freshener pads on your eyes and lie down on the slant board for 15 minutes. It'll do the trick every time.

Some Exercises for Traveling

Do you do a lot of traveling? Here are some exercises you can do while sitting in a car, bus, train or plane.

1. Tighten the tummy muscles to full tension. Hold for a count of five. Relax. Repeat ten times.
2. Raise one knee to a height of about eight inches above the other knee. Hold for a count of three. Relax. Repeat with the other knee. Alternate ten times.
3. To relieve tension in the lower back on a long trip, try this. Place both hands on the waist; bring the elbows forward as far as you can. Then move the elbows back as far as you can. Repeat ten times.
4. To relax the shoulders, raise them as high as you can. Hold for a count of five. Relax. Repeat ten times.

Exercises on the Job

When the office is empty and you have a free moment, use it to do a few figure exercises. All of these can be done from a seated position.

1. Slowly, raise one knee as high as you can, pulling it into the tummy. Hold for a count of five. Lower. Repeat with other knee. Alternate ten times. This is excellent *for the abdomen and the thighs.*
2. *For the bust and upper arms:* Stretch arms to the sides at shoulder level. Make big circles with the arms, pulling the shoulders back as you go. Keep this up through the count of twenty.
3. *For the legs and feet:* Slip off your shoes and stretch your legs out to full length with the toes pointed. Hold at tension for the count of five. Relax. Repeat ten times.

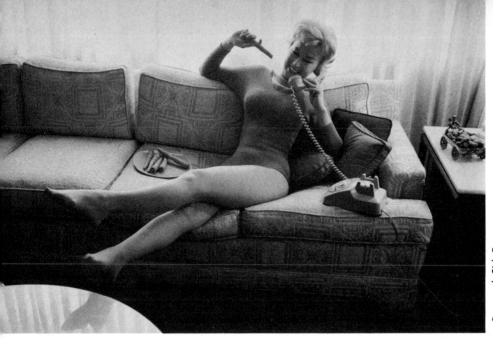

You can use time spent in telephoning to slim your
calves and thighs. Here I demonstrate the scissor kick.

4. *For the thighs and calves:* With the shoes off, move the
feet up and down on the toes twenty times.

While Telephoning

Clever girls never miss a chance to improve their figures.
Not even a telephone call can interrupt their beauty exercises.
Here are some easy ways to reduce the hips, thighs and knees
while you are gathering the local gossip.

1. While seated, extend the legs outward and do scissor
   kicks. Twenty times.
2. Cross the knees without letting one leg touch the other
   or letting the feet touch the floor. Alternate twenty
   times.

I think you can see from all of this how it is possible to
utilize many spare minutes during the day to do some simple
exercises that will supplement those you do at home. You'll
get in the habit of doing them whenever you can, which will
only make the road to perfection that much easier.

3

Figure Arithmetic

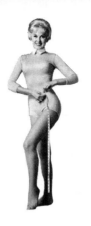

Adding, Subtracting and Dividing Your Weight

Let's find out how you measure up to the perfect proportions for your height and weight. Once we know how your weight is presently distributed, it is easy to shift it to the areas where it will be most attractive. Exercises will subtract unwanted inches from the hips, add them on to the bust, dividing the total body weight into its most appealing proportions.

You will need a tape measure, paper and pencil to record your measurements. Enter your findings on the chart at the end of this chapter or make an enlargement of this chart to hang over your mirror. In a few short weeks, you will be able to write in your new and improved measurements.

Start with the *bust:* Measure across the fullest part. Even if the measurements are satisfactory, you will want to do some exercises to lift and firm the bosom.

Next, measure the *waist:* This is easy to do if your waist is narrowed, for the tape will slip naturally into place. However, if you are overweight, you may have trouble determining your natural waistline. The waist should be measured at the point level with the elbows.

The *hips* should be measured at a point about seven inches down from the waistline.

The *thighs* are measured at the fullest part, just below the groin.

The *calves* are measured across the widest part, while standing barefoot.

The *ankles* are measured just above the ankle bone.

Fifteen minutes a day of figure exercises will bring you closer to your ideal measurements in just 30 days. Within 90 days, your measurements will approach your ideal goal.

The progress chart has a special section in which you may enter notes about your present muscle tone and tissue firmness. Check off the areas which need firming. As you slim and shape your body, you will be giving it youthful tone and tightening up the sagging areas.

If you are overweight or underweight, you will want to begin a new eating program for beauty, following the suggestions in the next two chapters. Proper diet adds or subtracts pounds. Exercise will divide your beauty weight into the right places, adding or subtracting inches. That is what I mean by Figure Arithmetic.

Check your weight at least once a week. At the first sign of an extra two pounds, nip the trend in the bud with a day of dieting to bring you back to your ideal weight. Overweight is easier to prevent than cure. Get rid of the first excess pound or two—and you will never have to worry about getting rid of any others. Once your weight is correct, you can keep it that way by eating at the rate of 15 calories per pound—which, you will find, is a generous daily quota—one that allows you to enjoy a wide variety of tasty foods.

Even though my own weight remains fairly stable, I like to go on a liquid diet for a full day every now and then, just to give my system an internal cleansing. This is an old Hollywood habit which many of the stars adopt just to give themselves a feeling of extra slenderness before they face the cameras.

By the time you reach your ideal proportions, I hope you will be so happy with the way your daily exercises make you look and feel that you will want to continue with them. Fifteen minutes a day of the Basic Six exercises which I outline in Part Two of this book will keep you perfectly proportioned and

In your program of figure beautification,
keep track of your measurements.
Check each week to note your improvement.

Ben and Sid Ross

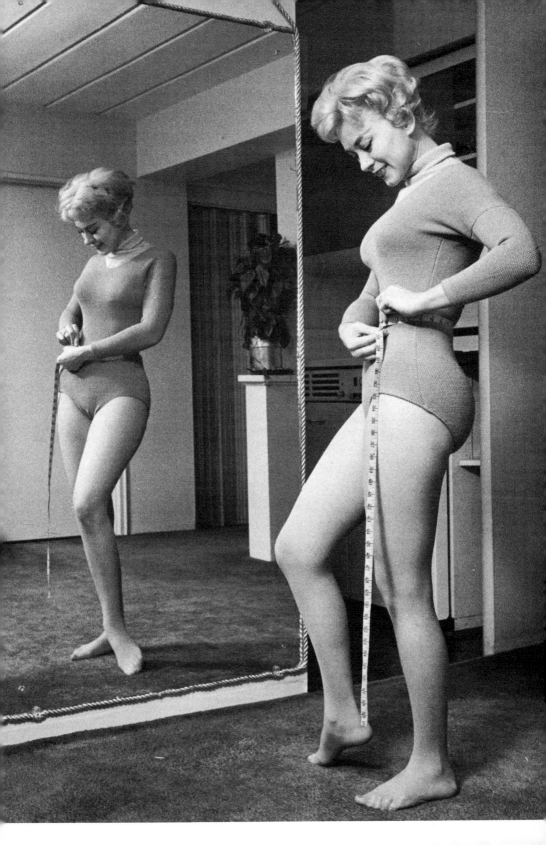

well-toned for the rest of your life. Measure yourself at least once a month—and if you note any tendency to gain or lose in any area, add a few special exercises to correct the problem before it becomes acute.

This simple maintenance program will keep your body youthful and attractive forever more.

What Shape Are You Wearing Today?

Our eyes often tell us what the scales, tape measure and pinch test fail to reveal. The female figure may be classified in six general shapes. Look at yourself from a distance in a full length mirror and let your eyes tell you in which outline your own figure seems to fit. Exercise will improve the silhouette and bring it closer to the ideal.

The Hourglass

The hourglass is the feminine ideal. The bust and hips are about the same in measurement. This is where your bone structure comes into play. A broad-shouldered girl can carry wider hips gracefully—whereas a smaller-boned girl cannot afford extra padding if she wants to keep her figure in attractive balance.

In the ideal figure, the waist should be from 10 to 12 inches smaller than the bust and hips. The waist may be even smaller, proportionately—depending on the body frame.

Whatever your present shape, you will soon bring it into hourglass proportions. Once you have achieved the ideal, you will want to know how to keep your pretty new figure at its best.

The Triangle

A small bust and heavy hips and thighs is the most common combination of figure faults. Don't be discouraged by your triangular proportions, however, for it is an easy matter to rearrange your weight to a more pleasing balance.

How to correct it: Check on your weight, first of all. Dieting will make it easier to bring those hips and thighs down to slender trimness.

Exercise will hasten the disappearance of extra inches in the lower torso—and build up an under-developed bustline. Start your fifteen-minutes-a-day with the Basic Six for general toning and proportioning. To these add 20 repetitions daily of the Finger Press and Wrist Clench to build up the bosom. Every other day, do additional bust-building exercises using weights. You can work up to a total of 30 repetitions for each of these exercises—but you should pause for 30 seconds to a minute between each ten repeats to get the best results. Books are usually sufficient weights for increasing, but you may use canned goods from your pantry shelf, if you prefer. A pair of household irons are ideal heavier weights but you should work up to using these gradually. Start off with the lighter weights and after six months you may advance to the heavier ones if your bust is unusually small.

The hips and thighs should get a generous share of your fifteen minutes. These reducing exercises may be done every day. As a rule, the hips go down more rapidly than the thighs. Therefore, it is a good idea to put your extra time into exercising for the thighs to hasten the slenderizing process.

If your waist is inclined to be thick, do at least 30 repetitions each of two waist exercises daily. You will be delighted to discover how quickly the waistline slims down. Just thirty days of exercising, along with your dieting, will bring forth rewarding results. If you are extremely overweight, it will take a little longer to reach your ideal measurements—but every two weeks will show exciting changes.

The Inverted Triangle

The inverted triangle is simply the triangle turned upside down. In this type of figure, the weight is concentrated on the upper half of the body—the hips are narrow and the legs slim.

But the waist, the bust, the upper arms and the back need reducing. Usually the tummy is in need of attention, too.

Many women who had good figures in their early years find
themselves slipping into this shape as they grow older. *Diet*
is a must to get rid of the extra pounds. Watch out for the
between-meal snacks. The extra calories settle down directly
in the waistline.

As the excess fat disappears with dieting, your exercises will
trim down the upper torso. Five minutes a day of exercises for
the upper arms and the back will make the bulges melt away.
Include a few specials for the Dowager's Hump, if you have
this problem. Give five minutes to the bustline every day, using
no weights—and the remaining five minutes to the waistline.
You may want to alternate this time schedule with a few
"lunges" and "squats" to build up the hips and thighs, if they
are too thin. Before you know it, you will be back to your
schoolgirl slenderness—looking just as pretty and young as
you once did.

The Oblong

Very thin girls might be called "oblongs." This was my problem in the teens. Appealing curves can be added by building
exercises.

If your weight is below normal, add a mid-morning serving
of toast and butter to your coffee break. A milk shake in the
afternoon will give you additional energy and add on the extra
pounds needed to fill in the curves. Pamper yourself with a
nap in the afternoon if you can possibly take one—and try to
get at least eight hours of sleep each night.

Exercise will keep the additional weight from settling in the
tummy and will put new roundness into the bust, hips and
thighs. Since the building exercises should be done only every
other day to be most effective, I suggest you do your bust-
building and hip-shaping on alternate days. This will give you
a chance to spend ten minutes on each—and leave five minutes
for the Basic Six every day.

One of the miracles of exercise is that many of the same
movements that slim down a full body will build up a thin one.

You exercise the muscles and they will adjust the contours to their most attractive proportions. Kick off your shoes and walk on your toes as often as possible to shape your legs if they are too thin. This takes no extra time and pays big beauty dividends.

The Round

The roly-polies are usually the shorter girls with delicate bone structure whose figures show every extra pound. Hollywood is full of could-be roly-polies who keep their glamorous figures by constant calorie-counting and daily exercise. Elizabeth Taylor and Carol Lynley are among the many famous beauties who fight a successful battle against the bulge.

Don't hide your pretty figure under a beauty-robbing blanket of fat. You probably just have a few pounds to lose—they merely look like more on a small frame. Thirty days of dieting will take away the excess pounds—safely and sensibly. Exercises will perfect the contours and firm the skin as your weight goes down.

The Square

A square figure is usually an athletic type of body which has gone overweight. The bone structure is more angular—square shoulders and a broader hip frame. A square figure becomes an ideal fashion figure when the weight is normalized. Jacqueline Kennedy is an example of the medium-framed athletic type. Her sleek proportions provide a perfect background for clothes. Ingrid Bergman is a beautiful example of the kind of figure perfection possible for women with larger body frames if they keep their weight and contours under control.

Most square figures are very solid. A reducing diet will make it easier for you to break down the hard layers of solid tissue with exercise. You can bounce away the fat on the hips and thighs, carve the waistline into trim, feminine slenderness and shave down the fullness of the back and upper arms with exercise. Five minutes a day on each of these areas will give you the lean, lithe contours that distinguish some of the world's leading beauties. Ankle and calf reducing exercises can be worked in during odd moments of your day, if your legs need some whittling down. Raise and lower yourself on your toes and rotate your ankles whenever you have a chance. You will be delighted at how well they respond.

Your Figure Dream Can Come True

Discover how easy it is to make any figure, regardless of its present problems, into an ideal figure. Don't for one minute believe that your problems are impossible to solve. When you see a beautiful movie star move gracefully across the screen, when you open a magazine and gaze with envy at the pictures of glamorous models, or simply pass an attractive woman on the street, don't ever think that their figures are one-in-a-million examples of accidental perfection. Your own figure can be just as perfect as those you envy if you decide to make it so.

It's easier to stick to a diet when you remember that every celebrity whose figure, as well as her face, is her fortune has to watch what she eats. Exercise is studio rule for famous figures. Cyd Charisse spends several hours a day on her dance routines—but still adds an extra period of other exercises to keep her fabulous figure well-proportioned. Ginger Rogers is an avid tennis player and golfer. Joan Crawford, Irene Dunne and Greer Garson owe their youthful bodies to self-discipline in their eating habits and daily exercise.

When you are tempted to give up a diet or skip your exercise routines—close your eyes for a moment and concentrate on the you that you would like to be—and can be—if you stick to your beauty program. It's not hard to pass up a piece of candy when you imagine yourself in a bathing suit. It's easy and fun to do a few toe touches every day when you picture yourself in a pair of slacks.

When the first five pounds disappear and the first two inches melt away, your own mirror will give you all the encouragement you need to continue with your diet and exercises. If you have a great deal of weight to lose, or much re-shaping to do, try thinking about it in smaller amounts. Work for those first five pounds and then go on to the next five. Attack your measurements inch by inch. Before you know it, your goal is reached! And every day you are growing younger and healthier —full of radiant vitality.

The time to begin your transformation is NOW. Try the Basic Six exercises on page 109 before you put this book down— and you will be on your way to an exciting new figure. Begin your beauty diet today by skipping dessert at your very next meal and choosing a piece of luscious ripe fruit instead. When you go to bed tonight, dream of the fun you are going to have with your glamorous new figure.

Why waste another day wishing for the figure that you want to have when you can be on your way to getting it just as easily?

The girls who did their exercises with me on television last spring are the ones who shone on the beaches last summer. The girls who exercised during the summer are the ones who are going to look their best in their new fall clothes. Those who begin in the fall are the ones who are going to give themselves the best Christmas present of all—a brand-new, beautiful figure! Any day is the right day to start on the easy path to beauty and health. Today is the very best day of all.

Your progress chart sets your goal for you. See for yourself how quickly you will achieve it. Soon your mirror and your friends will be complimenting you on your good looks and attractive figure.

YOUR IDEAL PROPORTIONS

Height (without shoes)	Bust	Waist	Hips	Thighs
4'8" 4'9"	31-33	20-22	31-33	17-18
4'10" 4'11" 5'	32-34	20-22	33-34	18-19

Height (without shoes)	Bust	Waist	Hips	Thighs
5'1" 5'2" 5'3"	34-35	21-23	34-35	19-20
5'4" 5'5" 5'6"	35-38	22-24	35-37	20-21
5'7" 5'8" 5'9"	36½-40	24-25½	36½-38	21-22
5'10" 5'11"	37½-41	25-27	37½-38½	22-23

(The variations allow for differences in bone structure. Check your body frame type by consulting the chart on the next page. Remember, the bust and hips should be the same; the waist 10 inches or more smaller than the bust and hips.)

PERSONAL PROGRESS CHECKLIST

	Start	30 Days	60 Days	90 Days	Ideal (your goal)
Height	—	—	—	—	—
Weight	—	—	—	—	—
Bust	—	—	—	—	—
Waist	—	—	—	—	—
Hips	—	—	—	—	—
Thighs	—	—	—	—	—
Calf	—	—	—	—	—
Ankles	—	—	—	—	—

Check the Areas Which Need Improving

Muscle tone and firmness

Bust_____   Abdomen_____   Outer Thighs_____   Arms_____

Waist_____   Hips_____   Inner Thighs_____   Back_____

Neckline_____   Others_____

Your Most Desirable Weight for Your Body Frame

Your frame type is determined by your wrist size. Measure the wrist at the joint between the wrist bone and the hand

	Wrist Size	Height
Small Frame	5½" or less	5'2" or under
	6" or less	5'3" to 5'4"
	6¼" or less	5'5" to 5'11"
Medium Frame	5½" to 5¾"	5'2" or under
	6" to 6¼"	5'3" to 5'4"
	6¼" to 6½"	5'5" to 5'11"
Large Frame	5¾" or more	5'2" or under
	6¼" or more	5'3" to 5'4"
	6½" or more	5'5" to 5'11"

IDEAL WEIGHT

Height (without shoes)	Small	Medium	Large
4'8"	92- 98	96-107	104-119
4'9"	94-101	98-110	106-122
4'10"	96-104	101-113	109-125
4'11"	99-107	104-116	112-128
5'	102-110	107-119	115-131

Height (without shoes)	Small	Medium	Large
5'1"	105-113	110-122	118-134
5'2"	108-116	113-126	121-138
5'3"	111-119	116-130	125-142
5'4"	114-123	120-135	129-146
5'5"	118-127	124-139	133-150
5'6"	122-131	128-143	137-154
5'7"	126-135	132-147	141-158
5'8"	130-140	136-151	145-161
5'9"	134-144	140-155	149-168
5'10"	138-148	144-159	153-173
5'11"	140-150	146-159	155-175

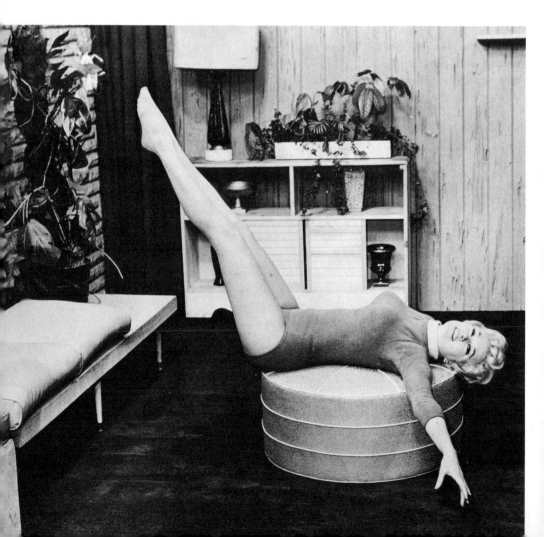

4

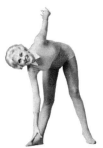

Eat Your Way to Health and Beauty

Real beauty—the kind that comes from a slender, healthy figure, a glowing, clear complexion, sparkling eyes, lustrous hair, strong white teeth—can't be purchased at cosmetic counters; it comes from the kinds of food you eat every day to keep your body at its natural best.

Good nutrition is the key to good looks, good spirits, a vigorous mind, and a long and happy life. But just what is good nutrition; how is it achieved? Briefly defined, good nutrition is an adequate supply of the food the body cells require for growth and maintenance, taken in a balanced proportion of the vital nutrients needed to sustain the life processes.

If certain elements are missing from the daily diet, the body breaks down in the same way an automobile ceases to run if it doesn't have a supply of gasoline and oil. The human body is made of protein, inside and out. Arteries, glands, muscles, connective tissue, skin, bones, hair, teeth, eyes—all contain protein and they need fresh supplies of protein to maintain, rebuild and repair themselves. Carbohydrates and fats produce energy. Vitamins and minerals are needed for the assimilation of food by the blood stream. Balanced nutrition means that the body is receiving a proper daily supply of these elements to give it strength, endurance and beauty.

Even your personality is dependent upon your daily diet. Lack of nutritional foods makes you tired, sluggish, dull. Your energy runs down, and your nerves are jumpy and on edge when you don't eat the foods that keep your body functioning at its best.

It's hard to believe—in this age of plenty—that anyone can suffer from malnutrition. Yet many people who eat three ample meals a day are "starving" themselves. They may be consuming generous quantities of food—even growing fat on what they eat—and still not be getting the life and beauty benefits their daily diets should offer them. They are eating what I call "food-less foods:" foods that lack the vitamin and mineral contents that provide youthful vitality.

You may be eating enough food to live, but how well are you living? To feel at your very best—to look your youngest and most beautiful—you need a balanced supply of the beauty builders every day.

To make sure that you are getting the most out of your daily food supply, check your present diet habits against this list of foods which doctors and nutritionists agree are the basic seven food groups. The amounts listed are the minimum daily requirements.

Eat These Foods Every Day

Meat, fish, poultry, cheese or eggs	1 to 2 servings
Milk (whole or skim)	2 glasses
Green, leafy vegetables	1 or more servings
Citrus fruits or tomatoes	1 or more servings
Other fruits and vegetables	1 or more servings
Bread, cereals (whole-grain or enriched)	2 slices of bread or 1 cup of cereal
Fat (butter or fortified margarine)	2 pats

You and your family can learn to eat the things that keep you young and healthy because they are *good,* not only because they are good *for* you. You've heard the old jest that everything attractive in life is either immoral, illegal or fattening. I will leave questions of morality up to the clergy, and legality up to the lawyers, but in the fields of diet and nutrition, which I have studied for years, I can say that the most nutritious foods are very often the tastiest.

A pleasant and satisfying conclusion to a meal need not include rich desserts. An accomplished hostess planning her most elegant dinner party may serve as a last course an attractive arrangement of fresh fruits or a fruit compote. These are nutritious and low in calorie count.

Drop That Sweet

Once you have lost the taste for sweets you will awaken to a whole new world of gastronomic delights; your palate will become sensitive to a whole new variety of taste treats. Just as a connoisseur of wine scorns the sweet, almost syrupy, muscatels and ports that are on the market, in favor of dry Burgundies or Bordeaux or Chablis, so can you educate your tastebuds to prefer natural foods to highly seasoned foods, tart foods to sweets, and broiled fish, fowl and meat to the fried variety.

If you are fond, for example, of fried fillet of sole or flounder, you don't know what you're missing until you have tasted a really well broiled flatfish, perhaps graced with a few paper-thin slices of almonds and a dash of paprika. Broiled fish is not only less fattening and more nutritious than fried fish, but broiling retains far more of the natural flavor than frying does.

I know of a small Scandinavian community on the shores of Lake Michigan, whose residents for many years have held weekly fish-fries at the beach on summer nights. But recently, because of the modern-day emphasis on nutrition and on a slim, healthy figure, they have given up their fish-fries, and turned them into fish-broils.

Those Vital Vitamins

Every part of our body requires nutrition—nutrition of a special kind. The bones require certain vitamins and minerals, the skin others, the liver others, and the circulatory system still others.

Later I will talk about vitamin supplements, but first let us look into the vitamins available in every-day foods. If we stick to the balanced diet based on the seven basic groups that I have listed we will absorb all of the basic vitamins required for good health. However, your doctor may be able to point out to you your own particular supplementary vitamin needs above and beyond what is recommended in my list.

Shop for as much variety as possible at the produce counters. You will make your meals more interesting and appetizing—as well as more nutritious—if you follow the simple guide of alternating your food choices wherever you can.

To give you a better idea of why varying your menus is wise, let me list the major vitamins and their richest natural sources.

VITAMIN A: This is often termed the beauty vitamin. Doctors measure its values not so much by what it will do for us as by what would happen if we were without it. A deficiency in vitamin A can produce skin disfigurations and vision defects. A is very important in building up the body's resistance to infections and disease. It benefits the eyes, the skin, the hair, the organs and the glands. My grandmother used to tell me to eat plenty of carrots if I wanted curly hair and a pretty complexion. I doubt that she had ever read about vitamins, but her instincts were certainly correct. Carrots are a rich source of vitamin A. Flyers discovered the importance of vitamin A in the prevention of night blindness.

Sources: Liver, kidneys, green leafy vegetables, cheese, eggs, tomatoes, spinach, carrots, peas, sweet potatoes, squash, dried apricots, whole milk, butter and fortified margarine.

VITAMIN B: The B's represent a whole family of vitamins. Most familiar to us are B_1, which is also called thiamine and B_2, known as riboflavin. Others in the group are niacin and the B complex vitamins. The B group is vital to our appetite and digestion, our nervous systems and our skin. Thiamine and riboflavin aid lactation.

Sources: Whole-grain breads and cereals, meats, fish, nuts, dried peas and beans, milk, eggs, fruits and vegetables.

VITAMIN C: Sometimes called ascorbic acid, vitamin C is highly important to the skin and tissues. A deficiency in vitamin C can cause spongy gums, skin degeneration and deterioration of the bones and joints. For smooth complexions, strong teeth and gums, youthful, firm body tissues—get your daily quota of vitamin C.

Sources: Citrus fruits, tomatoes and cabbage are important sources. Berries, melons, peppers, leafy green vegetables are valuable sources, too.

Vitamin D: Most mothers are familiar with the importance of vitamin D in preventing rickets in their children. D is the bone vitamin and is equally beneficial for the development of strong teeth. It helps the body utilize the calcium content of foods. The ultraviolet rays in sunshine are nature's gift of vitamin D. To make sure we get enough of this valuable vitamin, however, we must include the food sources in our diet.

Sources: Cod liver oil, egg yolks, Vitamin D-fortified milk.

Vitamin E: This vitamin does so many valuable things for the body that scientists are still adding to the list. It is known to be vital in preventing sterility and aiding the reproductive process. There is research being conducted now on the relationship of vitamin E to the prevention and cure of muscular dystrophy.

Sources: Wheat germ oil, whole-grain cereals, milk, butter, eggs and liver. Lettuce and other salad greens are good sources, too.

Vitamin Supplements

A balanced diet will guard you against possible vitamin deficiencies. However, to make up for the loss of some vitamins in food handling and processing, a multiple vitamin pill each day, following your doctor's advice, will assure you of your minimal needs.

As important as vitamins are to the maintenance of your health, it is quite possible to overdo a good thing. Never take extra doses of individual vitamins except under a doctor's guidance. The effect of overdosage can be a serious shock to your chemical balance. Ask your family physician to recommend a good multiple vitamin tablet. Do not experiment with other vitamin supplements on your own—no matter what miracle reports you may read about or hear from your friends.

Commercial vitamins are to be selected only under a doctor's advice. These pills vary: some are of organically grown components, extracted from their natural sources in foods. Others are synthetically composed in laboratories. The natural vitamins are more readily assimilated by the body than the synthetic types and are, therefore, preferable. It is your doctor who should make the specific recommendations.

Preserving Your Natural Vitamin Supply

Vine-ripened fruits and vegetables are richer in vitamin content than those which ripen after picking. Since many of our foods are shipped over long distances, it is necessary for growers to pick them before they are fully ripened to avoid spoilage in shipping. By the time they reach local grocery stores, they have lost many of their valuable vitamins. Overcooking, improper storage and handling in our kitchens is responsible for additional loss of vitamin value.

Commercial processing also involves a sacrifice in vitamins. Many canned fruits and vegetables are not as high in vitamin content as they were when they were freshly picked. Cooking and the use of artificial preservatives diminish the vitamin value.

You can do a great service to yourself and your family by handling your foods at home in a way that will make the most of their vitamin content. Here are some suggestions.

Eleven Easy Ways to Preserve Vitamins in Our Foods

1. *Serve fruits and vegetables as fresh as possible.* Each day of storage means a loss in nutritional values. Quick-freezing will preserve the vitamins better than ordinary storage.

2. *Prepare fruit juices immediately before serving.* Don't squeeze your citrus juices or mix frozen concentrates until you

are ready to drink them. If it is necessary to store them, be sure they are tightly covered and kept cold.

3. *Do not cut, peel or prepare vegetables until you are ready to use them.*

4. *Cook and serve your vegetables in their natural coverings whenever possible.* Many of the vitamin and mineral values are peeled away with the paring knife. Clean the skins well and serve the vegetables in Nature's jacket. Eat the baked potato skins. They have more food value than the inside portion.

5. *Cook frozen vegetables while they are still frozen.* Thawing them before cooking lets the vitamins escape.

6. *Keep foods tightly covered while cooking.* An open cooking pan allows the vitamins to escape into the air. A tight lid will seal them in.

7. *Do not overcook vegetables.* Limp vegetables mean the goodness has been cooked right out of them. Green vegetables are at their nutritious best when they retain their bright coloring. Serve your vegetables cooked through but somewhat resistant to the bite.

8. *Never use baking soda when cooking vegetables.* This is an old-fashioned method of preserving color used by some people. The addition of this soda destroys valuable vitamin content.

9. *Eat your fruits and vegetables raw as often as possible.* Cooking tends to lessen the food values. The only exception is if your doctor has a special reason for telling you to avoid raw foods.

10. *Use small amounts of water and raise the temperature rapidly when boiling vegetables.* The less water, the less dissipation of vitamins. The higher the temperature, the shorter the cooking time.

11. *Serve vegetables with their natural juices.* Don't pour the vitamins down the drain. The cooking water, also, can be used for sauces, soups and gravies.

Eat the Natural Way

Many of the so-called "refinements" of foods are actually health-stealers. The more natural the food, the greater the nutritional value. When flour is bleached, the greatest share of vitamins and minerals are removed from the grain. One hundred per cent whole-wheat bread, whole-grain cereals contain the natural nutrients. "Enriched" breads are those to which vitamins have been added to make up for those lost in the bleaching process.

Rice is another example of a nutritious, natural food that loses its life-giving values through processing. Brown rice retains the nutrients. Don't waste your money, your cooking time and your calories on polished rices.

Refined sugar contains no vitamins at all. The only sweetener I use is honey. I enjoy honey on my cereal, in my coffee and with fruits. While reducing, I use a saccharin sweetener—no food value here, either, but neither are there any calories.

Wheat germ is another favorite on my pantry shelf. It is nutritious food by itself, and makes an ideal topping for cereals or as a substitute for crumbs in the preparation of other dishes. It is nature's gift of concentrated vitamins.

Economize the Healthy Way

With rising costs and growing families to feed, there is often a great temptation to serve more starches (macaroni, spaghetti, noodles and rice) and less of the protein-rich foods than nutritional wisdom would call for. Your budget need not call for any sacrifice in nutritional value if you invest your food allowance in the items that give you the greatest health returns for your money.

Poultry and fish are less expensive than most meats and just as high in food value. You need not buy the most costly cuts of meat in order to get your proteins. Chopped beef is just as nutritious as a sirloin steak. A lamb stew is as nourishing as a lamb chop. Try to buy lean cuts of meat whenever possible. Trim away the fat before cooking your meats and use the natural juices as gravy. It's the meat that has the protein, not the fat.

The glandular meats such as liver, kidneys and lungs are rich sources of body-building materials. They are inexpensive treats to the gourmet palate when appetizingly prepared.

Cereals which you cook for yourself cost less per serving than the prepared types . . . and most of them have more food value.

Fortified margarine gives you as many nutritional benefits as butter and is far less expensive.

Skimmed milk is as nutritious as whole milk (and has fewer calories). When you mix your skimmed milk at home from non-fat crystals, it costs only a few cents a quart.

Fresh fruits and vegetables are the best investment you can make with your food dollars. Serve them lavishly when they are in season. You get the double advantage of buying them "home grown" which means less loss of vitamins—and they are less expensive than when they are imported from other regions. But don't skimp on them even when their prices go up—for they provide important protection against colds and infection.

The place where you can save real money on your budget is by cutting down on pies, pastries, cakes, doughnuts, cookies and other baked goods. These are made with bleached flour, refined sugar and oils that offer no contribution to your physical fitness. Doing without them benefits both your pocketbook and your health.

A Word About Water

Water by itself cannot be considered a food, but without water, foods cannot be digested. Water is vital to life in many ways: it cleanses, lubricates and aids in elimination of wastes.

Six to eight glasses of water a day are considered the necessary minimum by doctors and nutritionists. I always drink a glass of warm water first thing upon arising in the morning. If you add the juice of half a lemon to the water, you encourage natural regularity and add to your vitamin C intake. I keep a container of water in my refrigerator at all times. It is surprisingly tasty and refreshing and seems more thirst quenching than a glass of water drawn from the tap.

Anyone bothered by complexion problems will do well to increase her daily intake of water. It is just as important to wash the skin from within as from without.

Change Your Eating Habits
The Easy Way

Our eating habits are part of our daily living pattern. The way we shop, the way we cook, the way we serve our meals, the between-meal snacks, coffee breaks, the way we entertain —all are integral parts of our general daily life. To change these habits abruptly is very difficult for the average person.

To help you make this transition from "food-less foods" to a healthy eating pattern, I have devised a week-to-week plan which is simple to follow. It has worked wonders for me and for hundreds of others. Each change comes gradually. It is much easier to adopt one new habit at a time than to change all of your eating habits suddenly. At the end of the first week, you will have become accustomed to one new pattern in your eating. You will continue to follow this habit as you start with another one the next week. Within a few weeks, you will have made the changeover to nutritious, life-giving, health- and beauty-building ways of eating.

FIRST WEEK: This is your first step toward eating fresh fruits regularly. Every day for the first week, without fail, eat one of the following: an apple, an orange, a banana, a peach or a pear—or another fruit of your choice. Change from day to day to relieve the monotony.

SECOND WEEK: Eat one slice of 100% whole-wheat bread every day. Continue with your daily consumption of fresh fruit which, by now, you are accustomed to having.

THIRD WEEK: Drink two glasses of skimmed milk every day. Take it whenever you prefer—at meals, between meals, before retiring. But make sure you get your daily quota. Remember, too, that you are continuing the habits acquired during the first and second week.

FOURTH WEEK: Eat one raw vegetable every day. You may take it "straight" or mixed in a salad. Carrot and celery sticks can be taken as snacks or as part of your lunch or dinner. Lettuce, raw spinach, raw cauliflower, raw zucchini, cucumbers and tomatoes combine deliciously in salads. Raw mushrooms make ideal substitutes for before-meal appetizers. Experiment with a variety of vegetables. You will be surprised to find how tasty many of them are when eaten raw.

FIFTH WEEK: For dessert, have *only one* of the following each day: One scoop of sherbet; one serving of fruit (raw or cooked); one serving of baked fruit with honey (grapefruit is delicious this way); one serving of fruit gelatin. No other desserts this week. No pie, no cake, no pastry.

SIXTH WEEK: This week you will avoid all fried foods. Your eggs will be boiled or poached. Your meats will be broiled, baked, or boiled. You will lock up your frying pan for one entire week.

Without you or your family realizing it, you will have changed your entire style of eating in just six weeks. If you will stick to this new set of eating patterns, you will feel and look one hundred per cent better.

Other Health Habits

The week-by-week way to good health can also be applied to other habits which affect your appearance, your disposition and your general physical fitness. For one full week, dedicate yourself to getting eight full hours of sleep each night, if your system seems to require it. This is not hard to do just for one week. When you discover how much better you feel, you won't need any urging to make it another one of your lifetime habits.

Here's another tip on how to feel and look better. For one whole week, have a window wide open while you sleep and while you exercise. By the end of the week you will be so used to the idea that you will automatically keep it up.

5

Debbie's Easy Way to Reduce

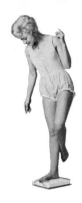

What does being overweight actually mean? Pick up a five-pound sack of sugar or a 25-pound sack of charcoal. Carry it around the room with you for a few minutes. Beginning to puff a little? It's a real burden. Yet the scales may tell you that you are carrying this much excess freight around with you, day in and day out. Imagine the pleasure—the relief—that could be yours if you threw off this excess baggage.

Don't fret about going on a diet. It's not all that difficult. Don't conjure up visions of yourself in perpetual hunger, despondently nibbling on tasteless wafers, desperately trying to resist the temptation offered by a dish of ice cream or a crisp waffle, smothered by maple syrup. With proper dieting you *won't* be hungry, and as the pounds melt away, you will begin to feel better than you have felt in years.

Face the Fats

There is no getting around the fact that what you eat is responsible for what you weigh, and unless you have a care for your calories, there may be no getting around *you*. Your body can use up only a certain amount of food each day. It takes what it needs from what you feed it, converts it into energy. What is left over goes into dead storage. This is where our friend the calorie comes into play. The calorie is a measuring stick. It is the term used to measure the energy value in foods. Each food has its own amount of energy value. To lose weight,

62

you should choose the foods that are tasty and nutritious, but have lower calorie counts than the fat-builders.

As a famous French writer once said, "Tell me what you eat, and I'll tell you what you are."

Try the Substitution System

Substitution—not starvation—is the key to successful reducing. Fill up on the foods that are low in calories; avoid the foods that are high in calories.

The easiest way to get started is to analyze your present eating habits. Do you have a pet indulgence that is responsible for overweight? Perhaps it is desserts—or between-meal snacks —or a weakness for potatoes and gravy. Maybe it's just the second helpings that overload your daily calorie count. Once you put your finger on your problem, you will know how to handle it.

If desserts are your temptation, by all means continue to have them. But substitute dietetic puddings, gelatins, or fresh water-packed canned fruits for your usual choices. Dress them up with non-fat whipped toppings and they will look just as inviting and taste just as good as the calorie-laden concoctions to which you have been addicted.

Between-meal snacks can be turned into beauty lifts instead of weight-lifts. For the mid-morning break, treat yourself to a half of a grapefruit or a slice of melon. In the afternoon, drink a glass of skim milk instead of a milk shake. Keep a supply of carrot and celery sticks in your refrigerator. They are just as satisfying as cheese and crackers and have only a fraction of the calories.

How to solve the potatoes and gravy passion? That's not as hard as it sounds. Simply broil the meat, use the natural juices for gravy, and bake the potato. Sprinkle chopped chives over the potato—or any other herb that you particularly like. Enjoy the crispy flavor of the jacket and soon you will wonder how you ever liked meat and potatoes any other way.

What can you do about the urge for second helpings? This is going to involve a little old-fashioned will power. Have your second helpings, by all means, but limit them to one at a meal and be sure the seconds are of salad, vegetable or fruit. Try this easy form of self-discipline for just a week. By then you will have little difficulty in saying no to the second helpings that are robbing you of your beauty.

Here are a few *positive* thoughts which have helped other women shed the pounds that kept them from having their full share of fun, laughter, and love:

> *I am going to live longer if I lose weight.* (Statistics will bear this out.)
>
> *I am going to be more popular when I have a good figure.* (A slim, attractive woman is always sought after.)
>
> *My husband is going to be proud of my new figure.* (All men admire a pretty, young-looking wife.)
>
> *I am going to feel better when I am at my correct weight.* (Many illnesses, aches, pains, chronic fatigue and general listlessness can be traced directly to overweight.)
>
> *I am going to look younger when I lose weight.* (Overweight adds years to your appearance. A slim figure is a young figure.)

Whenever you are tempted to "let go" and eat the things you know are bad for your figure, remind yourself of your goal. Take a good look at the tempting delicacy and ask yourself which you would rather have, that extra canapé (60 calories), that dish of ice cream (165 calories), that piece of candy (145 calories) OR a beautiful figure. If you are the bargain hunter I think you are, the choice will be very simple.

How to Count Your Calorie Needs

At the end of this chapter is a calorie chart. I hope you will study it until calorie-counting becomes second nature to you. Once you get in the habit of totaling up your daily count, you will have no trouble in sticking to a reducing plan.

When you know your calorie counts, you can actually set the date on which you will be 10 to 20 pounds lighter. The calories you cut out of your diet each day will determine your weight loss rate. If you are about average in your activities, your body requires about 15 calories a day for each pound of body weight. If your ideal weight is 135 pounds, you need about 2000 calories a day to maintain that weight. If you cut your present eating rate down to 1000 calories a day, your body will draw on stored fat for the other 1000 calories a day it needs for maintenance, and the result will be a loss of two pounds a week.

Proteins Help You to Reduce

High-protein diets are very effective for reducers. There are two reasons why proteins make losing weight easier. One is that proteins protect your body against weakness and fatigue. They keep you feeling energetic and strong even though you are eating fewer calories than usual. The other reason is that they speed the process of burning off the storage fats. The same calorie count in a high-protein diet will make you lose weight faster than that calorie quota in a low-protein diet.

Meats, fish, poultry, cheese and eggs are the richest sources of proteins. The egg is particularly beneficial in a reducing diet because its particular protein content hurries the burning-off process even more rapidly than other types of animal protein.

Unless your doctor has special reasons for counselling you to avoid a high-protein diet, I suggest you devote an ample share of your daily calories to foods which are high in protein content.

What About Starches and Sugars?

Your body is inclined to be lazy in making its selection of energy sources. It will always choose the easiest, quickest form of energy for its needs. Sugar converts directly into energy and your body will use up sugar before it turns to the energy contents in other foods. Next, it will select the starches. If you want to take weight off and are going on a reducing diet, it is wise to lower your intake of sugar and starches. For example, to fulfill your desire for a sweet beverage, why not try a high-quality low-calorie bottled drink. The body will then draw energy from your warehouse of stored fat which is what you want to get rid of.

All I Want Is the Fats, Ma'am

It is important to have a small amount of fat each day—even when you are reducing. Two pats of butter, as I have said, are the nutritional minimum. Any amount over this should be very limited when you are trying to lose weight. The minimum amount is all your body requires for lubrication. The rest goes into storage. The pats of today become the fats of tomorrow!

Salt contains no calories but it works to retain the water in the body tissues. Part of your weight loss is based upon eliminating the excess fluids in your system. If you use little or no salt on your foods, you will speed up the reducing process. Herbs make a delicious substitute for salt in seasoning. I have come to prefer them. I use them freely in cooking meats and vegetables and keep small containers of herbs on hand for table use.

What About Alcohol?

I don't drink because I don't care for liquor and find that I can get along just as well without it. But I recognize that a great many people do enjoy alcoholic beverages and that drinks are certainly to be considered in a reducing diet.

Alcoholic drinks of all kinds have a very high calorie count. If you put a share of your limited daily calories into liquor, it is obvious that you are going to have to subtract the equivalent amount from some other part of your diet—and this means sacrificing some of your nutritional needs.

You should plan to "go on the wagon" for the duration of your diet. Fruit or tomato juice, or bouillon on the "rocks" make agreeable substitutes for cocktails. They have far fewer calories to the glass than the 150 calories in a dry martini.

If you want to have an occasional cocktail or highball before dinner, just keep in mind the calories you will be adding.

Try to choose a drink with the lowest calorie count. You may discover it is just as satisfying as another with more calories. Alcoholic beverages tend to stimulate the appetite and thus you will eat more than you planned.

To prove my point, look at the calorie counts of these popular alcoholic beverages:

COCKTAILS (2 ozs.)		MIXED DRINKS (1½ ozs. liquor)	
Martini	150	Gin and tonic	125
Manhattan	175	Collins	175
Old Fashioned	200	Cuba Libre	200
Whiskey Sour	175	Tom and Jerry	225
Daiquiri	150	Eggnog	275
Vodka Martini	175	Vodka and Tonic	125

HIGHBALLS (1½ ozs. liquor)		WINES (3 ozs.)		BEER AND ALE (12 oz. can)	
Whiskey/Soda or Water (100 proof)	125	Dry red or white	75	Beer	170
Scotch/Soda or water (86 proof)	100	Sweet red or white	100	Ale	225
Whiskey/Ginger Ale	175	Sherry, dry	100		
		Sherry, sweet	150		
		Port	150		
		Dry vermouth	100		
		Sweet vermouth	175		

The Three Types of Overweight

There are three general types of overweight problems and each requires a slightly different reducing plan.

TYPE I—*If you are 25 pounds or more over your ideal weight,* you have a problem which may require medical attention. This type of obesity often arises from glandular malfunction. An underactive thyroid gland will keep your body from using the food fuels at a normal rate. Your body tends to store more food and get less energy from it. This type of glandular trouble makes you feel tired and sluggish most of the time. Your doctor can give you medication to restore the balance.

When the medical problem is solved, a reducing diet will get rid of the fat which your body has been storing in great quantities.

Obese persons with underactive thyroids have been accustomed to overeating for a long period of time. Their bodies crave the satisfaction and energy which food should provide, but their systems have not been able to make proper use of these foods. They eat more and more in an attempt to satisfy their needs. When the glandular balance is restored, they find it difficult to break the old eating patterns. Appetite is more of a habit than true hunger. There is a psychological longing for food, even when the body does not require it for its functions. It is this artificial hunger that must be curbed and that is a real test of character.

Obviously, the more weight you have to lose, the longer it is going to take to lose it. This may sound discouraging but there is a compensation for the very obese. If you have been used to seeing yourself as much as 50, 60 or 70 pounds overweight, you can look forward to a miraculous improvement in your entire appearance when your weight goes down.

The first ten pounds are the real struggle. When they disappear, you will know that success is possible and be encouraged to continue. You will have won the first round of battle with your old eating habits. The longer you can stay away from the old temptations, the more you become used to cutting down on quantities, the easier those habits become.

A "crash" diet which brings fast weight loss in a relatively short period of time is of little use to those who are greatly overweight. The greatest value of a crash program is psychological: quick results are encouraging as a reducing starter. The danger, however, is the temptation to stay on a crash diet for too long a time. You are eager to lose weight and the fastest way possible is the most appealing. It is important to realize that a crash diet is intended as a temporary eating pattern only. You should use the crash system for only three days at a time and no more than once a month, or it can lead to serious health disorders.

Stop for a moment and think how lucky you are. That may be hard to believe if you tip the scales at 200—but look at it this way. You are living at a time when more information, more help, more encouragements to reducing exist than ever before. Doctors can help you correct any medical problems that are causing your obesity. We know far more now than ever before in history what it takes to keep you physically fit and attractive. Think of all the people working to help YOU get the lovely figure you desire.

Don't Be a Scale Watcher!

When you start on a long-term weight reduction program, do not weigh yourself too frequently. Two weeks is the best interval between check-ups on the scales. The reason for this is that when you are making drastic changes in your system, there are bound to be day-to-day ups and downs. You may not lose rapidly in the beginning. Perhaps no change will show up for a full two weeks. If you are constantly checking your weight, you may become discouraged and feel that the diet isn't working. Give yourself enough time. Your doctor, I and everyone else who has made a study of reducing guarantee that you will lose weight if you stick to a low-calorie eating plan. Give your diet a chance to work for you.

Exercise is of double importance to you. Most fat people are "sitters." They are used to moving slowly and rarely engage in vigorous activities. Start to "think thin" and get in the habit of doing things that thin people do. Exercise will help you develop the bodily grace that goes with your new figure. You must follow a daily exercise routine to get your figure into proper proportion as your weight goes down. When you lose a large amount of weight, you may be left with stretch marks and sagging skin unless you tone the muscles. Exercise will make your body young and firm as your weight goes down. Do more walking. Try your hand at active sports. I have often thought that one of the reasons fat women don't engage in sports activities very much is that they are ashamed to be seen in sports clothes that reveal more of the figure. Pretty soon, *you* are going to have a figure that looks well in shorts, bathing

suits and slacks. Start learning some sports skills now to be
ready for your new future.

Your reducing diet should allow for no more than 1500 calories a day (unless your doctor specifies otherwise). If you can
bring this total down to 1000 or 1250, so much the better. You
may expect to lose from five to ten pounds a month on this
type of calorie plan.

Make Up for Your Lapses

Become an expert on calorie counts. Study the charts at the
end of chapter four. Buy a pocket size calorie counter and keep
it in your handbag. Check the calorie count before buying your
groceries or ordering in a restaurant. Keep a notebook with you
to record your caloric intake each day. The more you remind
yourself of your diet, the easier it will be to lose weight.

TYPE II—*If you are 10 pounds to 25 pounds overweight,*
your problem is not quite as extreme as Type I. However, the
shorter you are, the more noticeable—and the more dangerous
—your extra weight is. Why not get busy from this moment on
to bring your weight down to its ideal level?

If you have gained this extra weight within a relatively short
period of time (a year or less), you had better check with your
doctor. The rapid gain may be due to a health problem which
he can readily detect and remedy. Then go on a reducing plan
to get rid of the extra pounds.

More often, this kind of weight sneaks up on a woman. If
she has gained too much weight during pregnancy, she is apt
to keep it after the baby is born. Many young married women
get trapped by this situation. They overeat during pregnancy
(the old-fashioned idea of eating for two is plain nonsense. The
mother feeds herself healthfully and moderately and Nature
takes care of feeding the baby). If the new mother nurses her
baby, she eats abundantly to keep up her milk supply. (This is
all too often overdone, too.) By the time the baby is weaned,
the mother is in the habit of overeating. She often becomes
pregnant again and the cycle resumes. Within a few years, she

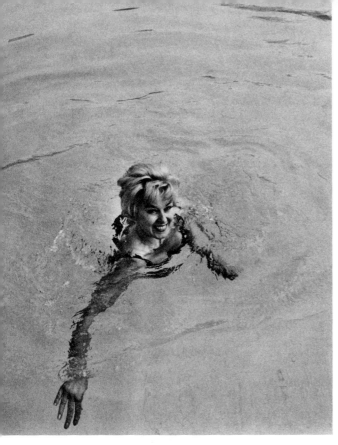

Whenever possible I like to supplement my daily stint of exercise with a brisk swim. Swimming is one of the best all-around conditioners. But if you have to lose weight, don't neglect calorie-counting.

has gone up, up, up in weight and is desperate about her lost figure.

Middle age is another danger period for weight gain. We used to think that it was healthy to put on a little weight with the years. Doctors have thrown out all these ideas now. They state that one's weight at 25 is the weight which should be maintained throughout life. Since it is a natural tendency to decrease activity with age, the diet that maintained weight at 25 becomes a weight-gaining diet in later years. We should all learn to eat less and less as we grow older. Daily exercise will keep the body firm, shapely and youthful.

The glandular changes that occur in the middle years are often responsible for an increase in weight. This, again, is the "creeping" kind of gain. The pounds come on, one by one, and the woman doesn't realize what is happening until she wakes up one morning and her mirror tells her she is the victim of the middle-aged spread. The additional weight usually settles in the waistline, stomach and hip girdle. But don't let anyone fool you into believing that gaining weight is inevitable and that nothing can be done about it. Consistent exercise and moderate eating patterns can prevent it. Even when the problem has actually occurred, it can be cured by diet and exercise. Youthful proportions can be yours at any age.

The time it will take to bring your figure back to attractive proportions depends upon how much weight you have to lose. Ten pounds can disappear in thirty days or less. More reduction will take proportionately longer. Your best diet plan is based upon 1200 calories a day. This will usually get rid of 10 to 15 pounds in a month to six weeks. If you are 15 to 25 pounds overweight, a 1500 calorie plan is preferable. It takes a little longer but your weight is more apt to remain stable when you have reached your ideal level.

TYPE III—*If you are less than 10 pounds overweight,* you should have no difficulty at all in shedding the extra fat. This is the most usual form of overweight. Even when your weight falls near the desirable level for your height, the mirror will often indicate the need for reducing. Doctors tell us it is safer to be a few pounds underweight than over. If you want to streamline your figure, you will want to get rid of the extra pounds and work hard on your exercises to get yourself into perfect shape.

It is up to you to choose the road that is easiest for you to follow. By all means, experiment with my quick, crash diets (with your doctor's approval)—but make up your mind to the fact that you cannot stay on them for more than three days at a time and can use them only once a month. When you reach your ideal level, continue to curb your caloric intake and learn to live without the fattening foods that are responsible for your gaining tendencies. With your pretty new figure to encourage you, this shouldn't be hard to do.

The better way, by far, to lose those few extra pounds and keep a perfect figure forever is to start out on a consistent, nutritiously-balanced lower-calorie diet and let the extra pounds slip away gradually. This is your assurance that they will never return.

10 Easy Ways to Cut Down on Calories

1. Eat your meals as usual but cut the quantities in half.

2. Eliminate *all* between-meal nibbling. (This takes real fortitude but it will be easier if you remember that snacks are one of the major causes of overweight.)

3. Start your meals with clear soup or bouillon. It will curb your appetite.

4. Increase the bulk whenever possible. You will get more satisfaction without adding calories. Whole fruits fill you up more than the same amount in juices. Watermelon is one of my favorite bulky fruits. Puffed cereals are more filling than flakes.

5. Avoid all desserts except fresh or stewed fruits.

6. Avoid bread and butter with lunch and dinner.

7. Eat no fried foods of any kind.

8. Add no milk, cream or sugar to coffee or tea.

9. Plan your meals well in advance, using a calorie chart to guide your selections.

10. Stock your pantry with low-calorie, dietetic foods.

Any one of these ten tips will help you lose weight. The more of them you adopt, the faster you will reduce.

How to Make Dieting Easier

Eat slowly: Any amount of food seems like more when you eat it slowly. Cut your food into small pieces and chew them carefully. Pick up smaller portions with your fork or spoon than you normally do each time. Studies have shown that fast eaters are more inclined to overweight than those who eat slowly.

Serve your meals attractively: The more you satisfy your eye, the more you will satisfy your hunger. Even if you eat alone, prepare each meal as though it were a special occasion. Use garnishes of parsley with your meats. Decorate serving platters with curls of carrots, radishes, green peppers. Cut your morning toast into four triangles. Slice roasted meats paper-thin. The same amount will look like more if it is thinly sliced. Choose your vegetables with an eye for color to make a pleasing picture on your plate.

Spark up your mealtime conversation: Search for interesting subjects and save them for mealtime discussion. If your conversation is lively, you will have fewer thoughts to spare for food.

Take up a new hobby: If you find new spheres of interest, you will not think about food as much.

Don't talk about your diet: Your family and close friends will want to know what is going on—but generally speaking, the less said about your diet, the better. Rather, let the results speak for themselves. Strangely enough some people seem to urge food upon you when they know you are dieting. A polite "no, thank you" is more effective than a prolonged discussion of your diet.

Find a symbol for your goal: This can work wonders. Pin up a photograph of the bathing suit you would like to wear. Put your "before" picture alongside a picture of a girl with the kind of figure you would like to have. Resolve not to buy one new article of clothing until you can buy it in a smaller size.

Celebrate your success: Pick your first weight loss goal (five or ten pounds)—and when you have lost that amount, celebrate! Not with a trip to the soda fountain, but with a special movie, concert or outing. Or buy yourself a bottle of perfume— anything that seems a special reward to you.

Low Calorie Foods

To get you off to the right start in your low-calorie thinking, here is a list of foods that are full of nutritional value but low in calories. This will give you some idea of the variety possible in your reducing menus.

MEAT, FISH AND POULTRY: (You may have two servings a day of these, but don't fry them.)

Lean Beef	Liver or Kidney	Halibut
Lean Lamb	Crabmeat	Haddock
Lean Veal	Lobster	Brook Trout
Chicken	Codfish	Sole
Turkey	Oysters	Whitefish
Pork Chops, fat removed		Salmon, not canned

EGGS: 1 or 2 a day

Poached or Boiled. Hard-boiled eggs have more bulk; are, therefore, more satisfying.
Scrambled without butter

VEGETABLES: Raw or cooked. You may have 3 servings daily
of these, more, if you like. Serve them without butter, sauces
or dressings. Season with herbs and use their natural juices for
gravy.

Artichokes	Chard	Parsley
Asparagus	Cucumbers	Radishes
Beets	Endive	Romaine
Beet Greens	Escarole	Spinach
Brussels Sprouts	Green Beans	Summer Squash
Broccoli	Green Peppers	Tomatoes
Cabbage	Lettuce	Turnips
Carrots	Mushrooms	Wax Beans
Cauliflower	Okra	Zucchini
Celery		

CITRUS FRUITS: (At least 1 a day)

Lemons	Grapefruit	Tangerines
Limes	Oranges	

OTHER FRUITS: (At least 1 serving a day)

Apple	Cantaloupe	Plums
Apricots	Cherries	Raspberries
Blueberries	Grapes	Strawberries
Blackberries	Peaches	Watermelon

DAIRY PRODUCTS:

Buttermilk, 2 glasses a day
Skim milk, 2 glasses a day
Cottage cheese, ½ cup a day, instead of meat occasionally

BREAD AND CEREALS: (2 slices or 1 cup a day)

Enriched white bread	40% Bran flakes	Cream of Wheat
100% whole-wheat bread	Oatmeal	Wheatena
All-Bran	Farina	Wheat flakes

FATS: (2 pats daily)

Butter
Fortified Margarine

EXTRAS ALLOWED:

Black coffee	Low calorie, dietetic	Low calorie
Plain tea	salad dressing,	beverage,1 glass
	1 tablespoon	Low calorie gelatin
	Dietetic jelly or	dessert,1 serving
	jam, 1 teaspoon	

If you stick to these low calorie foods in the amounts specified, you will lose weight quickly and safely without having to
keep a special calorie count.

High Protein Diet Plan

A high protein diet maintains your energy at top level and
hastens the reducing process. When following this type of diet,
it is important to eat all of the foods specified as they create a
chemical combination that burns off the extra fat. Do not eat
anything other than the foods prescribed. Choose your meats,
fish, poultry, fruits and vegetables from the general low-calorie
list on the previous pages.

Do not prepare your foods with fats or oils of any kind. Use
only saccharin sweeteners. On the third day, you may add the
extras listed in the low-calorie group—but take no more than
the amounts specified.

If you stick to this plan, you can expect to lose an average of
a pound a day. The diet plan includes all of the Basic Seven
foods to give you balanced nutrition. Let me caution you about
following a high protein diet if you have high blood pressure,
kidney trouble or hardening of the arteries. Consult your doctor for his approval before starting a high protein diet.

BREAKFAST

Citrus fruit (1 orange or ½ grapefruit. Take the whole
    fruit rather than the juice for greater bulk satisfaction)
Egg (1 or 2) boiled, poached, or scrambled without butter
Bread (½ slice whole wheat bread with 1 pat butter or
    margarine)
Coffee or tea (without cream or sugar)
Skim milk (½ glass)

LUNCH

Meat, Fish or Fowl (Trim off the fat; broil, bake or boil)
Cooked vegetable or salad (No butter, no dressing)
Fruit (Fresh or dietetic canned. One teaspoon of honey as
    sweetener, if desired)
Skimmed milk or buttermilk (1 glass)
Coffee or tea (Without cream or sugar)

DINNER

Meat, Fish or Fowl (Trim off the fat. Bake, broil or boil)
Vegetable
Fruit (1 teaspoon of honey as sweetener, if desired)
Skimmed milk (1 glass)
Coffee or tea (No cream or sugar)
(American or cottage cheese may be used in place of meat,
    fish or fowl)

900 Calorie Plan

For quick and healthy weight reduction, here is a 900 calorie
a day plan which gives you freedom of choice in composing
your own menus. Keep the Basic Seven in mind as you make
your selections, however, to make sure you are getting all you
need for balanced nutrition.

Breakfast: Select 300 calories from the following:

	Calories		Calories
½ medium orange	25	½ cup corn flakes	50
½ grapefruit	50	6 oz.-glass whole milk	125
3 cooked prunes	75	6 oz.-glass skim milk	75
1 teaspoon butter	50	½ tablespoon heavy cream	25
½ cup oatmeal	75	1 teaspoon sugar	25
½ cup Cream of Wheat	75	1 egg	75
1 slice whole-wheat bread	75	1 saltine	20
4 oz.-glass tomato juice	25	black coffee, plain tea	0

Lunch: Select 300 calories from the following:

6 stalks of asparagus	20	¾ cup cooked cabbage	25
½ cup Brussels sprouts	30	½ cup eggplant	25
3 stalks of celery	15	2 small green peppers	25
10 slices cucumber	15	1 cup green beans	25
½ head of lettuce	35	1 small tomato	20
½ cup cooked spinach	15	¾ cup carrots	30
½ cup canned tuna	100	¾ cup turnips	25
½ cup canned salmon	80	1 small apple	55
¼ cup cottage cheese	25	½ cantaloupe	40
1 egg	75	black coffee, plain tea	0
1 slice whole-wheat bread	75	6 oz.-glass skim milk	75

Dinner: Select 300 calories from the following:

1 cup vegetable soup	80	2 slices roast veal	200
1 cup spinach soup	80	1 slice roast chicken	50
1 cup beet soup	80	½ small broiled chicken	100
1 slice lean roast beef	100	1 egg	75
2 lean hamburger patties	200	1 small piece broiled haddock	50
1 portion round steak	100	6 large oysters	60
1 slice roast lamb	100	1 piece brook trout	50
1 slice whole-wheat bread	75	black coffee, plain tea	0

Appetite bonus: if you want to increase your daily caloric intake to 1200 calories, you can do so by adding on to this basic 900 calorie plan. You will not lose as rapidly but you will lose—and safely!

Crash Diets

I use these two crash diets when I have splurged and want to bring my weight back down to normal in a hurry. Never stay on either of these diets for more than three days at a time and do not repeat them more than once a month. There is not enough variety of life-giving foods to supply the system with its required nutritional needs.

Supplement any crash diet with a multiple vitamin pill each day.

Debbie's Quick Reducers

1. Breakfast, lunch and dinner are the same. No substitutes, no extras allowed.
   ¾ cup cottage cheese on lettuce
   1 banana
   1 glass of skim milk
   black coffee or plain tea (saccharin sweetener, if desired)

2. Breakfast, lunch and dinner are the same. No substitutes, no extras allowed.
   1 cup of whole-wheat or bran cereal
   1 teaspoon of honey
   I glass of skim milk
   black coffee or plain tea (saccharin sweetener, if desired)

You can see for yourself why I caution you about continuing these diets for more than three days. However, I doubt, determined as you may be to lose weight, that you would have the heart to face this fare for a longer period anyhow. I know I wouldn't!

The Foods Concentrate Plans

One of the more recent inventions in reducing diets is the food concentrate plan. This plan is based on a pre-mixed food which can be purchased in liquid form or as a dry powder to which water is added. This type of diet is based on 900 calories a day, spread over the three meals. The concentrate is supposed to contain a balanced assortment of foods, minerals and vitamins to cover all the nutritional requirements.

I have experimented with these concentrates and found that they do take the weight off as promised. However, this diet does not have much visual or taste appeal—though it does satisfy the appetite. The plan is valuable when used as a single meal substitute, rather than for three meals a day. Rather than eat a quick meal that is not balanced nutritionally, you are better off to substitute a 300 calorie allotment of the concentrate.

One great disadvantage of the 900 calorie concentrate plan is that it does not teach you anything about counting calories for yourself. When you drop this diet, your weight will go right back to where it was unless you follow a continuing calorie control plan in your everyday eating.

If you have only a pound or two to lose, this is a quick and easy way to lose it. If you have a larger amount of weight to lose, I suggest you check with your doctor and get his advice on how best you might use this new reducing food.

Don't Skip Meals

One more word to add to the subject of weight reduction. Starvation is *not* the answer to reducing. When you skip a meal, it only means that you will eat more at the next meal to make up for it. Feast and famine dieting will keep your weight on a constant elevator ride and seriously endanger your health.

Going for long periods without eating can result in disturbances of the body balance. When you do not put anything into your stomach for a long period of time, you deny your system what it requires to neutralize the stomach acids. This may result in extreme stomach irritation, indigestion—even ulcers.

By the same token, excessively large meals are dangerous. When you overload your stomach at one meal, you cause an excessive burden on the heart and the digestive tract. This pulls the blood away from the brain and creates mental and physical lethargy. If that heavy meal is taken prior to bedtime, it encourages weight gain. The body, while sleeping, is able to absorb a higher percentage of carbohydrates as it does not require them for fuel when inactive. The food goes directly into fat—usually lodging in the stomach, waist and hips.

Reducing—like any self-improvement endeavor—is based upon mental attitude. The body is equipped to cope with the lesser amounts of food and still function healthfully and normally in every respect. The mental and emotional reactions to a reducing diet are the most difficult hurdles to overcome. You can fortify yourself for the change in your eating patterns . . . try making up your mind which is most important to you: a serving of pie or cake; a special gourmet sauce; nibbles and snacks; a cocktail—or a beautiful, healthy, slender figure.

The Problem of Underweight

Adding weight is just as difficult for some women as losing it is for others. Extreme thinness may be due to glandular deficiency. If the thyroid gland is overactive, the body burns off all its food supply leaving a minimum supply of fat to build up the tissues.

If your weight is more than five per cent below the ideal level for your height, you should consult your doctor to determine if there is a medical cause involved. If you are an active person and a naturally "picky" eater, you can help yourself develop a more attractive figure by reversing some of the principles applied to reducing plans.

Eat more and worry less are the two best rules for building up weight. Your weight often indicates your emotional structure. The skinny types are usually the ones who burn off their calories with nervous energy. To gain weight, you must learn to slow down a little. Get as much rest as possible—"forty winks" after mealtimes will give your system a chance to absorb the food. Eight hours of sleep each night should be your regular minimum. Ten hours are even better.

If you are on a weight-gaining diet, it does not mean indiscriminate choice of foods. There are many healthful foods which are also high in calories. The chart below will give many suggestions to help you plan well-balanced meals which include foods with a high count. You may find between-meal and bedtime snacks a pleasant way to add calories.

To gain weight, I suggest that you try a week-by-week plan to slowly change over your eating habits. Try adding just 100 calories to your regular fare each day for one week. The following week, add another 100 calories (a total of 200 daily). Stay on the 200 extra calorie plan for two full weeks and check in with your scale. If you are not adding the necessary pounds, you may have to add more to your daily diet.

Exercise serves two valuable purposes for the thin figure. It helps to stimulate the appetite AND it builds up curves. Fifteen minutes a day of my exercise for body building will increase your shapeliness.

CALORIE CHART

(Based on studies by the U.S. Department of Agriculture)

MILK AND MILK PRODUCTS:	Amount	Calories
Whole milk	1 cup (8 ozs.)	165
Skimmed milk	1 cup (8 ozs.)	90
Buttermilk	1 cup (8 ozs.)	90
Cream, light	1 tablespoon	30
Cream, heavy	1 tablespoon	50
Yoghurt	1 cup	120
Cheese:		
Cheddar or American	1 ounce	115
Cottage, skim milk	1 ounce	25
Cottage, creamed	1 ounce	30
Roquefort, or Blue	1 ounce	105
Swiss	1 ounce	105
Desserts:		
Cornstarch pudding	1 cup	275
Baked custard	1 cup	285
Ice Cream	1 serving	165

EGGS:	Amount	Calories
Whole	1	75
Boiled or poached	1	75
Fried or Scrambled	1	110

MEAT AND POULTRY:	Amount	Calories
Bacon, medium crisp	2 slices	95
Beef:		
Pot roast, lean only	1 slice	115
with fat	1 slice	340
Hamburger, regular grind	1 patty	245
lean round	1 patty	185
Roast, prime rib, lean only	1 slice	110
with fat	1 slice	350
Steak, lean only	3-ounce portion	105
with fat	3-ounce portion	375
Corned beef,	3 ounces	180
canned hash	3 ounces	120
Beef stew, with vegetables	1 cup	250
Chicken:		
Broiled	½ small broiler	115
Roasted	2 slices	100
Fried	½ small fryer	350
Lamb:		
Chops, lean only	1 chop	130
with fat	1 chop	450
Roast leg, lean only	1 slice	120
with fat	1 slice	265
Shoulder, lean only	3 ounces	125
with fat	3 ounces	300
Liver: (Beef or Calves)		
Fried	2 ounces	120
Pork:		
Chops, lean only	1 chop	120
with fat	1 chop	340
Roast, lean only	1 slice (3 ozs.)	160
with fat	1 slice	340

	Amount	Calories
Ham: (Cured, Smoked)		
Baked	1 slice	340
Boiled	1 slice	170
Spiced luncheon meat	1 slice	165
Tongue: (Beef)		
Boiled or Simmered	3 ounces	205
Veal:		
Cutlet, broiled	3 ounces	185
Roast, lean	3 ounces	185

FISH AND SHELLFISH:	Amount	Calories
Bluefish, baked or broiled	3 ounces	135
Clams, raw	6	100
Crabmeat	3 ounces	90
Fishsticks, breaded	1	40
Haddock, fried	3 ounces	135
Mackerel, broiled	3 ounces	200
canned	3 ounces	155
Oysters, raw	6	60
stew	1 cup	200
Salmon, baked or broiled	1 steak	200
canned	3 ounces	120
loaf	1 slice	225
Shrimp, fresh or dry pack	6	100
Sardines, canned	3 ounces	180
Swordfish, broiled	½ steak	150

DRY BEANS, NUTS:	Amount	Calories
Beans, canned		
red	1 cup	230
white, with pork	1 cup	330
without pork	1 cup	315
limas (dried) cooked	1 cup	260
Cashews, roasted	1 cup	770
Peanuts, roasted, shelled	1 cup	840
Peanut butter	1 tablespoon	90
Walnuts, shelled	1 cup	750

VEGETABLES:

	Amount	Calories
Asparagus	6 spears	20
Beans		
lima	1 cup	150
string	1 cup	25
Beets	1 cup	70
Broccoli	1 cup	70
Cabbage, raw, shredded	1 cup	25
cooked	1 cup	40
Carrots, raw	1 whole	20
cooked	1 cup	45
Cauliflower	1 cup	30
Celery	1 stalk	30
Corn, fresh	1 ear	65
canned	1 cup	170
Cucumbers	6 slices	5
Endive	2 ounces	10
Escarole	2 ounces	10
Lettuce	4 leaves	5
	1 small head	70
Mushrooms, fresh	12	25
canned	1 cup	30
Onions, raw	1 medium	50
Peas, green		
fresh	1 cup	110
canned	1 cup	170
Peppers, green	1 medium	15
Potatoes, Baked	1 medium	90
Boiled	1 medium	90
Chips	10	110
French Fried		
frozen	10 pieces	95
home-fried	10 pieces	155
Mashed	1 cup	230
Radishes	4 small	10
Sauerkraut, canned	1 cup	30
Spinach, cooked	1 cup	45
Squash, Summer	1 cup	35
Squash, Winter	1 cup	96
Sweet potatoes, baked	1 medium	155
boiled	1 medium	170
candied	1 small	295
canned	1 cup	235
Tomatoes, raw	1 medium	30
canned	1 cup	45
juice	1 cup	50

FRUITS:	Amount	Calories
Apples, raw	1 medium	70
juice	1 cup	125
sauce, sweetened	1 cup	185
unsweetened	1 cup	100
Apricots, raw	3	55
canned,		
heavy syrup	1 cup	200
water pack	1 cup	80
Apricots, dried	10	100
cooked	1 cup	240
Avocados, California	1 whole	370
Bananas	1 medium	85
Blueberries, raw	1 cup	85
Cantaloupes	½ melon	40
Dates	1 cup	505
Fruit cocktail, canned	1 cup	175
Grapefruit, raw	½	50
canned, syrup	1 cup	165
water pack	1 cup	70
juice	1 cup	96
Grapes	1 cup	70
Grape juice, canned	1 cup	165
Lemon juice, fresh	1 cup	60
Oranges, fresh	1 large	70
juice	1 cup	105
Peaches, raw	1 medium	35
canned, syrup	1 cup	185
water pack	1 cup	65
Pears, raw	1	100
canned syrup	1 cup	175
Pineapple, raw	1 cup	75
canned, crushed	1 cup	205
canned, sliced	1 large	95
juice	1 cup	120
Prunes, dried		
uncooked	4 medium	70
cooked	1 cup	295
juice	1 cup	170
Raisins	1 cup	460
Strawberries, fresh	1 cup	55
frozen	1 cup	240
Watermelon	1 wedge (4" x 8")	120

BREADS, ROLLS & CEREALS:	Amount	Calories
Hot Breads:		
Bran muffins	1	125
Cinnamon buns	1	150
Coffee cake	1 piece	100
Cornmeal muffins	1	100
English muffins	1	100
Waffles	1	250
Breads:		
Rye	1 slice	55-70
White	1 slice	60-75
Whole-Wheat	1 slice	55-70
Cereals:		
Bran flakes	½ cup	75
Corn flakes	½ cup	50
Oatmeal, cooked	½ cup	75
Farina, cooked	½ cup	55
Shredded wheat	1 biscuit	100
Wheat germ	1 tablespoon	15

DESSERTS:	Amount	Calories
Apple brown betty	1 cup	350
Bread pudding	1 cup	500
Chocolate pudding	1 cup	400
Cream puffs, filled	1	150
Custard	1 cup	285
Doughnuts	1	150
Eclairs, filled	1	300
Gelatin plain, unsweetened	1 teaspoon	10
fruit flavored	1 cup	125
Pies, average	1 wedge	approx. 350

FATS & OILS:	Amount	Calories
Butter	1 tablespoon	100
Cooking fats, vegetable	1 tablespoon	110
lard	1 tablespoon	125

FATS & OILS (Cont.):	Amount	Calories
Margarine	1 tablespoon	100
Oils, salad or cooking	1 tablespoon	125
Salad dressings		
Blue cheese	1 tablespoon	90
French	1 tablespoon	60
Mayonnaise	1 tablespoon	100
Russian	1 tablespoon	75

SUGARS, SWEETS:	Amount	Calories
Candy, average type	1 piece	approx. 125
Chocolate syrup	1 tablespoon	40
Honey	1 tablespoon	60
Jams	1 tablespoon	55
Jellies	1 tablespoon	50
Sugar, granulated	1 tablespoon	50

MISCELLANEOUS:	Amount	Calories
Macaroni, plain	1 cup	175
with cheese	1 cup	475
Noodles	1 cup	200
Rice	1 cup	200
Spaghetti	1 cup	155
White sauce	1 cup	430

SOUPS:	Amount	Calories
Bean soup	1 cup	190
Beef soup	1 cup	100
Bouillon	1 cup	10
Consommé	1 cup	10
Chicken soup	1 cup	75
Cream soups	1 cup	200
Noodle, rice or barley	1 cup	115
Tomato	1 cup	90
Vegetable	1 cup	80

6

Especially for Teen-agers

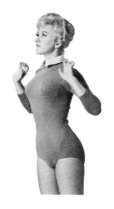

If you are in your teens or are the mother, relative or friend of a teen-ager this chapter is especially for you.

It is never too early to begin developing a trim, attractive, feminine figure. The girl who learns to control her weight during her teens will know how to stay slender for the rest of her life. The girl who exercises for perfect proportions in her early years will have an easy time keeping those measurements forever.

No teen-ager has to waste her tears or her time envying another girl's slim figure. Instead, she can work to make her own figure attractive. The sooner she begins, the longer she will be able to enjoy the self-confidence, poise and happiness that comes from knowing that she is at her best. Her growing body can be made to grow more beautiful and perfect each year. The guides for figure control which you find in the rest of this book apply just as much to teens as to women of other ages. There are, however, a few special factors about the teen years that should be taken into consideration.

The most important difference between the teens and the later years is growth. Between the ages of twelve and twenty the body undergoes changes of great significance. These changes are often upsetting to the sensitive adolescent for the body leaps upward (and often outward, too) in sudden spurts. There are no set rules about when these changes take place. One girl may grow several inches taller between the ages of thirteen and fifteen. Another girl may grow very gradually in her early teens and suddenly stretch upward as late as her sixteenth or seventeenth year. Teens often think they are "freaks" because they are shorter or taller than the other girls of their age. As long as they recognize the fact that these growing rates, however unpredictable, are entirely normal, they won't be upset. It is not until about the age of eighteen or even later that the figure fully develops. Of course there are exceptions. But again, this is entirely dependent upon each girl's individual growing rate. Some teens develop much earlier than others. A girl of fourteen may have already acquired a mature bustline. Another will not show any marked development in this area until her later teens. The measurements which I outline on my proportion chart are not usually possible for a girl to achieve in her early teens.

Exercises for Teen-agers

All of the exercises in Part Two can be used by teen-agers. A girl in her teens should identify her figure problems just as an older woman does, and choose the exercises especially designed to correct them.

One difference between a young bulge and an older one is in its firmness. Teen-age tissues are naturally firm and it takes an extra measure of exercise to reduce these solid areas. A teen-ager with heavy thighs or well-padded hips should do more of the "bouncing" exercises. Firm fat needs extra pounding to break it down. The more strenuous the exercises, the quicker the slimming process.

Unless a young teen-ager shows a decided tendency toward a heavy bosom, I recommend the bust-building exercises with weights every other day. An early start in developing the pectoral muscles will assure her of a firm, rounded bosom. The alternating hot and cold massages which I have described are especially beneficial in building the bustline if they are started in the early teens.

A teen-ager with a large bust should spend five minutes a day on decreasing and firming exercises to control the development and keep the bosom youthful.

Other special problems such as fat arms, thick calves and heavy ankles can be corrected more easily in the teens than in later years. Concentrated area exercises will make miraculous improvements.

Girls with average figures can perfect their contours by following a well-rounded routine of bust, waist, tummy, hip and thigh exercises. In just a month or two, it is possible to take an inch off the waist and add it on to the bust.

Tight foundation garments and binding brassieres should be avoided in the formative years. Exercise will enable a girl to achieve natural control, and from then on, a lightweight girdle and well-fitted bra are all she will need.

Sports Activities

As much as active sports contribute to a teen's all-around trimness and physical fitness, they will not replace the value of planned exercise in shaping the figure. These beauty exercises, as I like to call them, work directly upon the muscles and tissues to improve and feminize the contours. Sports activities improve the general muscle tone, burn off extra energy and at the same time give a girl the chance to inhale energizing fresh air. They are both important, but each serves a special purpose.

I consider swimming the best sports exercise for the figure. It develops the bust, slims the hips, tapers the legs and limbers the waist. Bicycling is another sport that provides beauty dividends for the figure.

Social dancing is one of the most enjoyable and, at the same time, most effective forms of exercise. While it does not fall into the sports category, the kind of dancing most teens do is active enough to put it under this heading. Such dancing is excellent for the figure and it develops bodily grace as well as attractive contours.

Ideal Weights for Teens

The ideal weights listed in Chapter 3 are for women 25 years of age and over. As a general rule, the weight during the teens should be about one pound less for each year under the ideal for that height at twenty-five. The accompanying chart lists average weights for teens by height and age.

WEIGHT CHART FOR TEEN-AGE GIRLS

Height	12 yrs.	13 yrs.	14 yrs.	15 yrs.	16 yrs.	17 yrs.	18 yrs.
4'2"	62 lbs.						
4'3"	65						
4'4"	67						
4'5"	69	71					
4'6"	71	73					
4'7"	75	77	78				
4'8"	79	81	83				
4'9"	82	84	88	92			
4'10"	86	88	93	96	101		
4'11"	90	92	96	100	103	104	
5'	95	97	101	105	108	109	111
5'1"	100	101	105	108	112	113	116
5'2"	105	106	109	113	115	117	118
5'3"	110	110	112	116	117	119	120
5'4"	114	115	117	119	120	122	123
5'5"		120	121	122	123	125	126
5'6"		124	124	125	128	129	130
5'7"		128	130	131	133	133	135
5'8"		131	133	135	136	138	138
5'9"			135	137	138	140	142
5'10"			136	138	140	142	144
5'11"			138	140	142	144	145

(Compiled by the Metropolitan Life Insurance Company)

Reducing Guides for Teens

Too often, well-meaning friends and families tell a teen-ager: "Don't worry about your weight—it's only baby fat and you'll grow out of it." This kind of advice may be good for the ego but it isn't going to do anything for a girl's figure. When the scales and the mirror tell a girl that she is over-weight, the kindest thing she can do for herself is to get rid of the extra pounds; she should give herself the slim figure that will make her happy and poised during her teens. She will have more pep, look prettier, wear clothes more attractively and have much more fun when she is slender and shapely.

Any diet for the teen years must be based upon extremely sound nutritional principles. Proteins are of special importance as they provide the body-building materials needed for growth. There is a great need for an ample supply of vitamins B and C in the early teens. This means plenty of orange juice, tomatoes, salads and vegetables. A reducing diet should in-

It's never too early to begin developing a trim, feminine figure. These young girls are learning principles of exercise and weight control that will keep them slim and attractive throughout their lives.

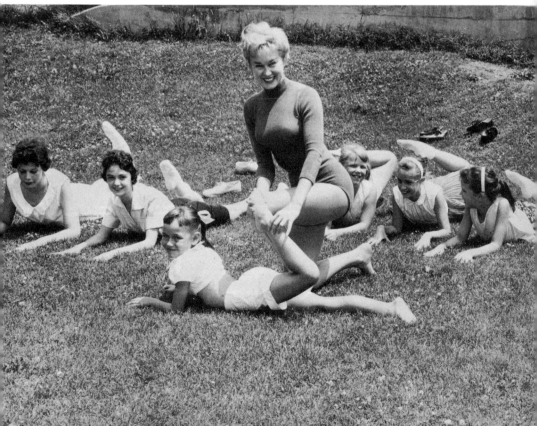

clude the basic foods listed in Chapter 4 to assure normal growth.

Between the ages of thirteen and fifteen, a girl has her greatest daily energy needs. 2600 calories a day is the generally accepted maintenance average. From the age of sixteen through nineteen, 2400 calories a day are recommended. These rates, of course, apply to a girl of normal weight. To reduce, the daily calorie intake must be cut below the maintenance level. A teenager should consult her doctor to find out what the same minimum level is for her individual body requirements and activity pattern.

Overweight in the teen years is caused by the same factor as overweight at any other age: overeating. The extra calories make the extra bulges. For instance, if you increase your calorie count by 100 each day, you can probably expect to gain ten pounds of weight in one year. As I have stressed in Chapter 5, successful reducing is based upon foregoing the extra little fatbuilders that are not essential to good nutrition, but simply build up the reservoirs of added pounds.

A doctor will probably recommend a daily calorie cut of 500 to 1000 calories from the present total. These calories can be taken out easily by cutting down on the snacks and sweets. A teen won't find it hard to make these small sacrifices if she realizes how important her new figure will be to her happiness. It's the fattening extras that are stealing her popularity by spoiling her figure.

Adolescent Complexion Problems

Adolescent skin problems usually have their roots in eating habits. The following foods have been termed "skin poisons" by doctors. Blemishes will clear up more rapidly if these foods are avoided:

| Nuts | Gravy | Carbonated beverages |
| Olive oil | Heavy cream | Doughnuts |

| Chocolate | Candy | French fries |
| Soda | Pastries | Fried foods of any kind |

To keep the complexion fresh and clear, a teen should eat an extra quantity of fresh fruits. Oranges, lemons and grapefruit are especially helpful. Tomatoes, green vegetables and skim milk are excellent for the skin. Water is an inside cleansing agent. Six to eight glasses of water a day will help to wash away the impurities that clog the pores and cause blemishes.

A Brief Word About Posture

Although I have emphasized the importance of good posture before, I feel it is a subject of special concern to teen-agers. Most posture problems begin in the teens. Up to the age of twelve, girls carry themselves with natural grace. But, somehow, from the age of thirteen, the slump begins.

Standing TALL is the first rule of figure beauty. Even though a girl is growing at what she may consider an alarming rate (often much faster than the boys in her class), humping her shoulders and drooping her head is not going to cut off the extra inches. A slump doesn't make a girl shorter—it only makes her unattractive.

Little girls have an obvious advantage in carrying themselves at full height. They give the impression of being taller than they actually are. Plump girls look slimmer and thin girls look more shapely when they carry themselves gracefully.

When carrying school books or any heavy bundles, the weight should be divided between the two arms. The constant pressure of books resting on one hip can lower that hip permanently. The tummy should be kept tightened and pulled in at all times, whether sitting, standing or walking.

Choose a Partner

Working with a partner on a figure-improvement plan makes exercising twice as much fun and dieting twice as easy.

My sister and I have been exercising together for over five years. At sixteen she has one of the best figures I have ever seen. We often turn on the phonograph and do our exercises to music. When she brings out her rock-and-roll records, fifteen minutes fly by in no time as we stretch and bend.

A mother-and-daughter team is ideal. Together they can design menus and prepare meals that are appetizing, nourishing and low in calories. A reducing diet is always easier to follow when another member of the family shares the same food restrictions. Exercising is a game when two can do it together.

A teen can have fun going into beauty-partnership with a school friend. Instead of stopping at the drug store for an after-school snack (which only adds more pounds), they can go to each other's houses to exercise. If each girl keeps a record of her weight and measurements, they can compare notes every month. The one who has made the most improvement in a thirty day period wins and can get a present from her partner. Two girls I know made life size figure silhouettes of themselves and tacked them to the walls of their rooms. Each week they would stand inside their old outlines and see how much they had "shrunk" from their former sizes.

Teens—Have the Figure
You Want—and Keep It

Weight and proportion control in the teens brings immediate benefits at a time when a girl is most self-conscious and concerned about her personal appearance. These benefits carry over for the rest of her life. If a girl's weight is normal in her teens, she will be less apt to gain weight after she marries and has children. If she is in the habit of exercising in her adolescent years, she will find it easier to continue her fifteen-minutes-a-day program as she grows older.

"As the twig is bent, so grows the tree." A teen's figure is in her own hands. She can start now to make it figure-perfect.

Teen Weight Chart

GIRLS

	13	14	15	16	17	18
4'5"	71					
4'6"	73					
4'7"	77	78				
4'8"	81	83				
4'9"	84	88	92			
4'10"	88	93	96	101		
4'11"	92	96	100	103	104	
5'	97	101	105	108	109	111
5'1"	101	105	108	112	113	116
5'2"	106	109	113	115	117	118
5'3"	110	112	116	117	119	120
5'4"	115	117	119	120	122	123
5'5"	120	121	122	123	125	126
5'6"	124	124	125	128	129	130
5'7"	128	130	131	133	133	135
5'8"	131	133	135	136	138	138
5'9"		135	137	138	140	142
5'10"		136	138	140	142	144
5'11"		138	140	142	144	145

7

It's Never Too Late to Begin

One of the most inspiring examples of figure improvement is that of Eleanor Powell. Miss Powell retired from motion pictures to devote herself to her husband and family. Like many another housewife and mother, she neglected her figure. She gave up the exercises that had kept her dancing figure well-proportioned. She put on weight. Then, in her forties, came a chance for a comeback. She was offered a contract to star in a Las Vegas hotel *if* she could get herself ready in time. It was a frightening challenge. So much to do—to *un*-do—in a short time. But she met the challenge. She lost over 30 pounds and exercised vigorously every day until she regained her dancing figure. When the big night of the opening came, she was ready, and the audience cheered a young, vivacious, beautiful Eleanor Powell as it had twenty years before.

If you think your age makes it impossible for you to have a good figure, remind yourself of Eleanor Powell who turned back the clock—and the many other stars who have defied the turn of the calendar pages to prove that a woman can remain eternally young if she takes good care of her body.

The advantage a mature woman has over her juniors in building a beautiful figure is that time endows her with greater powers of self-control and self-discipline. Youth is impatient, impetuous. Time teaches patience, forbearance. She learns by experience that good things are worth working and waiting for.

When you understand the year by year transitions of the body, you are better equipped to combat the ravages of time and take the necessary steps to restore and maintain its natural perfection.

In your twenties, your body begins to lose its natural elasticity, unless you keep exercising the muscles. If neglected, the proportions begin to change. The most common tendency is for the bust to decrease in size and firmness—and the hips and thighs to increase in girth. The tissues start to soften. The inner thighs loosen and a general sagging of the skin gets under way.

The reasons for these changes are both circumstantial and self-imposed. You tend to follow fewer sports activities than you did in the teen years. If you have a job, you are probably sitting down most of the time. Your hips can increase as much as three inches and your bustline decrease as much as two inches without any change in your weight. A few minutes a day of planned exercise will prevent these changes.

If you get married, you tend to change your eating habits. As a new bride you are anxious to please your husband with your cooking skills. You prepare many special dishes to please him—and they are usually filled with extra calories. If you eat as much as your husband does, the results soon show on the scales. You should eat only two-thirds as much as he does. The same number of calories that maintain a man's weight increase a woman's weight because of the difference in body frame sizes.

The next challenge to your figure comes along with the babies. Too often, pregnancy is used as an excuse for overeating. The baby takes only as much nourishment from the mother as it requires. The excess calories turn to fat and make it more difficult to get your figure back to normal after the baby is born. Diet control and daily exercises during pregnancy will keep you in better health, make delivery easier and assure you of regaining your slender figure. If your doctor approves, I recommend the resumption of planned exercise three days after childbirth. This will restore the muscle tone and hasten the return of the organs to their original positions. But please check with your doctor, first.

If you have neglected your figure during your twenties, the thirties only bring an increase in proportion problems. With the forties comes the change in bodily function that often brings with it a change in glandular balance and body contour. These changes can be the source of great frustration and emotional upset. However, they need not destroy your youthful figure if you do something about them. A doctor can give you remedies to correct the glandular imbalance. Diet and exercise will maintain the proportions. Any sudden tendency to lose or gain weight at this time should be noted and quickly reported to your doctor. "Middle-age spread" is not inevitable. It can be prevented or corrected by your eating habits and my easy fifteen minutes a day planned exercise program.

Many of the backaches, headaches, feelings of fatigue and other physical disturbances that prevail in the middle years can be attributed to overweight and under-exercise. The body wants to function properly, but nine times out of ten we fail to help it along.

How often have you heard someone say when they stoop to pick up something from the floor, "Oh, listen to my bones crack, guess I'm getting old." It is a mistake to believe that these things must happen as you grow older. What makes the body stiffen and age is not time, but neglect.

You know what happens to a lock that hasn't been used in many years. It gets rusty. When you put a key into it, it creaks and groans. The same thing happens to the joints of the body when they are inactive. They creak and groan, too. You oil the lock to make it usable again. Exercise is the "oil" the body joints need to remove the rust and get them into smooth working condition.

The same principle applies to the muscles. If you haven't bowled in twenty years, your arm muscles will ache after your first game. If you haven't been doing body exercises, the first few waist bends or leg raises will make you a little stiff. You can restore the muscle tone but it takes time to recondition the long-neglected parts of the body.

Bicycling is lots of fun as well as an excellent conditioner at any age. Moreover, the whole family can enjoy it together.

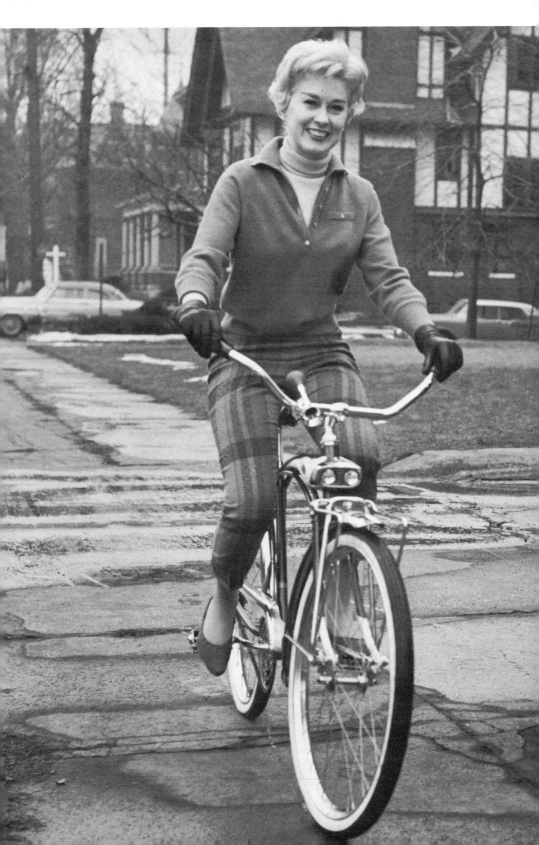

That is why I stress the importance of working up gradually to your full exercise routine. The Basic Six exercises are the easiest ways to get you started without unpleasant after-effects. For the first three days, do only six exercises and do them only five times each. After these three days, add one additional repetition until you reach fifteen counts. By the beginning of the second week, you are ready to add more exercises to your routine. These you will select to correct special figure problems. Start slowly with each new exercise. Remember that each new movement calls upon a new set of muscles and they must be accustomed to the action. The decreasing exercises can eventually be done up to twenty-five to forty-five times each!

Diet Habits
in the Maturing Years

Twenty-five is the age on which the desirable weight chart is based. Doctors tell us that your best weight at this age is the weight you should maintain for the rest of your life.

The old-fashioned idea of gaining a few pounds over the years as you grow older has been proven wrong. In fact, doctors now say that it is actually healthier to *lose* a few pounds rather than to gain them.

Even if you want only to maintain your weight—neither gain nor lose—it is important to cut down on your daily caloric intake as you get older. The body does not use up as much food as the years advance. The growing process has stopped and the extra calories are no longer needed. Each year you should be eating less rather than more. If you keep a close check on your weight, you can stop any gains before they get out of hand.

Constipation is a frequent problem in middle age. Your daily exercises will prove of great help in restoring normal regularity. Diet habits can keep your elimination regulated without the need for artificial aids. Drink plenty of water every day. Take your first glass immediately upon arising. Add the juice of half a lemon to encourage regularity. Watermelon or other melons are also beneficial. They flush the kidneys and guard against the swelling that accompanies constipation. Cooked prunes and apricots are excellent natural laxatives. So are figs, raisins and bran cereals. A decrease in your salt intake is helpful. I firmly believe you should try all the *natural* methods of improving regularity before resorting to patent medicines.

Let me caution you about the use of mineral oil. You should not use it in the preparation of food (frying, salad dressings, etc.) because it prevents the absorption of certain vitamins, as well as of calcium and phosphorous.

Special Exercises for the Mature Years

One of the best and easiest exercises for the mature years is s-t-r-e-t-c-h-i-n-g. A good stretch pulls the muscles and limbers them. Get in the habit of stretching hard and often as you get older.

Tummy tensing is another simple corrective exercise for older women. Pull the tummy muscles in and hold them for a count of five, relax and repeat. Do this often to restore firmness to a sagging stomach.

Get the kinks out of the spine with this exercise "massage." Sit on the floor and bring the knees up to the tummy. Clasp the knees firmly with your arms and roll backwards on your spine—all the way up to the shoulders. Roll up and down several times. This will relax the tension in the lower back and relieve the nerve centers along the spine.

An easy way to maintain muscle tone is by giving yourself a brisk towel massage after your bath or shower. Grasp the opposite ends of your bath towel and rub it briskly back and forth across the back. You can do the same thing on the thighs and legs. Give your feet a towel treat, too. Rub the towel back and forth across the arches.

You're as Young
as Your Breathing!

Deep breathing comes naturally to youngsters. The older you get, the shorter the breaths. The huffing and puffing we associate with "getting old" are the results of taking smaller and smaller amounts of air into the lungs with each breath.

To renew the youthful characteristics of deep breathing which keep the voice firm and resonant, practice these simple exercises:

1. Pant like a dog. Part your lips and breathe in and out rapidly. Repeat often.
2. Through the nose, take a small sniff. Hold the air and take a larger sniff. Hold again and take another larger sniff. Repeat until the lungs are full of air. Release all the air at once. Repeat often.
3. Stand in front of an open window and take in a large breath of fresh air. Hold the air in the lungs for a moment or two. Release. Repeat several times daily.

I was hospitalized for several weeks after a rather serious automobile accident. When I got out of the hospital and returned to my television show, I found that I had a great deal of difficulty in controlling my breathing. I ran out of breath easily and had a problem in talking during my exercises. I used these three breathing exercises regularly, repeating them several times each day, and within two weeks had recovered my breathing control.

You Are Never Too Old to Exercise

Some of my favorite students are ladies in their seventies. I have several who exercise along with each of my television shows and who send me periodic reports about their figure improvements. I have worked with many ladies in this age bracket in my studio experiences and find that they can take all the vigorous exercises which the younger girls do, provided their doctors issue no special cautions because of other health ailments. I think that a woman should be proud of her femininity and her figure throughout her life. Ruth St. Denis, the famous dancer, is an ardent devotee of exercise even though she proudly admits to being in her eighties. And she has a figure that many a teen-ager would envy! Exercise is not intended solely for the very young—exercise is the means of *keeping* you young!

8

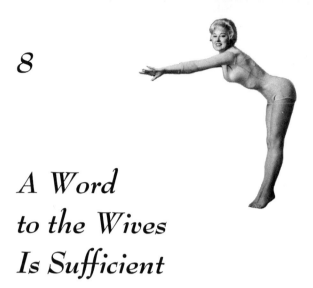

A Word
to the Wives
Is Sufficient

If the bloom seems to be disappearing from your marriage, your figure may be partially to blame! If you can still zip up your wedding dress after ten, fifteen or more years of marriage, you are much more likely to be keeping the honeymoon glow alive than if you have let your figure go.

Your physical appearance has a great deal to do with your marital happiness. The problem is two-sided. If you are self-conscious about figure imperfections, you have probably lost confidence in your powers of appeal. Secondly, the loss of youthful physical attractiveness has a decided psychological effect upon your husband. A man reacts quickly to his wife's lack of interest in her appearance. He believes it indicates an "I don't care" attitude and his romantic illusions begin to fade.

When you determine to improve your personal appearance and physical vitality, your husband's ego is bound to be inflated. He will interpret your efforts to be as appealing as possible as an attempt to please him and hold his affection. He will be flattered by your desire to attract him—and the romantic spark will be rekindled.

To keep your marriage fresh and exciting, you should do all you can to keep yourself youthful and vital. Your husband's eyes are not going to roam elsewhere when the prettiest girl he knows is home waiting for him. A balanced diet and regular exercise have far-reaching effects upon your marriage. Sound nutritional habits not only keep your weight at its most attractive level, assuring you a slim, pretty figure—but they also increase your general vitality. The Basic Seven foods provide a balance of vitamins and minerals which are nature's "pep" pills. They keep your body vigorous and energetic. Good eating habits keep you "internally young" as well as youthfully appealing.

As the "Chief Executive" of the kitchen department, you have a wonderful opportunity to select, prepare and serve the foods that will keep you and your husband healthy and zestful. Remember the old saying, "The way to a man's heart is through his stomach?" How very true—but not in the way grandmother interpreted the phrase. We know now that over-feeding your husband will tax his heart and sap his vitality. There are so many interesting ways that you can dress up the foods that maintain your husband's health, keep his weight down and yet intrigue his appetite. Brush his meats with taste-tantalizing herbs before putting them under the broiler—instead of into the frying pan. Cut a variety of fresh fruits into a chilled bowl and top them with low-calorie make-believe "whipped cream." Surprise him with tasty, filling casseroles that combine lean meats and vegetables instead of starches. He'll tell the world he married a great cook and you'll have the satisfaction of knowing that you are helping him stay healthy and youthfully slim.

Learning to Relax Together

Tension is the most dangerous enemy your marriage can have. Your husband brings home his business worries, financial burdens and daytime strains, and finds it difficult to put aside these problems when the day is over. After a busy day of housework, caring for the children, community projects and perhaps a job of your own, you find it just as hard to relax. These tensions build up and up—and destroy the happiness you used to find with each other. You can make these tensions disappear through the magic of exercise!

Try this plan some evening soon—and see for yourself what a soothing, relaxing effect it has upon both of you:

First of all, pamper your tired man with a head massage. Get him to sit down on the couch, perhaps when he is watching television, and rub his head with a gentle, but firm, rotating motion of your fingers. Start at the nape of the neck and work towards the forehead.

Before retiring, suggest that he try these "relaxercises" with you:

1. Stand with the feet slightly apart. Bend over at the waist and let the head and arms drop forward. Shake the head and shoulders, keeping them as loose as possible. Shake the arms, too. After several good shakes, pull the body up again to a standing position, letting the spine roll up in a lazy, relaxed motion. Repeat several times.

2. Sit on the floor with legs apart. Touch the right leg with the head. Straighten and touch the left leg with the head. Make the movements as elastic as possible to stretch the spine from the neck all the way down to the lower back. Repeat at least ten times.

3. Stand with the feet together. Take a deep breath and rise up on the toes. Hold the breath while remaining on tiptoes—then slowly exhale while coming down on the feet again. Repeat ten times.

If you each follow these relaxercises with a warm tub bath, you will go to bed with all the tensions gone and awaken the next morning with renewed vigor.

Part Two

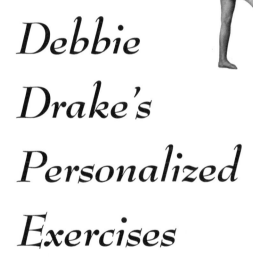

Debbie

Drake's

Personalized

Exercises

9

Six Sure Steps
to a Perfect Figure

Exercising every day is the key to achieving and keeping the attractive contours and youthful firmness that distinguish a perfect figure. Every woman, regardless of her age, weight and figure problems (or perfections) should do at least one exercise every day for the bust, waist, hips and thighs, tummy, upper arms and neckline. Exercising for figure beauty should be as much of your normal daily routine as cleansing your face and brushing your teeth.

Even if you are one of the rare women blessed with perfect proportions, you cannot preserve them unless you keep the muscle tone conditioned. Daily exercise is as necessary for maintaining a good figure as it is for acquiring one. Perfect figures don't happen by accident. They are the direct result of health habits. Hollywood stars, models and others whose figure beauty is vital to their success never skip a day of exercise. Every woman should follow a regular program of figure care if she wants to maintain her youthful contours.

If you are on a reducing diet, beauty exercises are a "must." Only through exercise can you sculpture your new body weight to the proportions which you desire. Losing weight is not enough to create a perfect figure. When a woman is overweight, the skin has been stretched and pulled to cover the excess fat. When the fat disappears as a result of dieting, the skin tissues hang loosely over the body. Think of a girdle that has been stretched to full size through continual wear—until it no longer returns to its original firm shape. The same principle applies to the skin tissues when they have been stretched out by overweight. The skin has lost its elasticity and cannot snap back to its original firmness when the support of fat has been removed. Exercise is the only means of restoring the skin's elasticity. Therefore, daily exercising is a vital accompaniment to a reducing diet.

Another word about exercise in connection with weight reduction. Heavy women have built up strong, unyielding areas of fatty tissue. In many cases, these lumps are very firm and solid. Exercises like the hip bounce, bicycling while lying on the side are designed to break down these resisting pads of hard tissue. All of my exercises will help improve the circulation and aid the body in carrying off the excess fat from these areas.

Exercise is just as important to those who are trying to gain weight. Thin figures need to build up the muscles and tissues which fill out curves. When you increase the caloric intake for weight gain, the extra pounds are apt to settle directly in the stomach. Exercise will enable you to put the extra weight where you want it—to fill out the bosom, shape the arms and legs.

The following six exercises have been carefully chosen to provide a basic beauty program for all women—regardless of individual figure differences. In the other chapters that follow, I will show you special exercises for various figure faults. These are to be used *in addition* to the BASIC SIX.

The BASIC SIX are to be done whether you are overweight, underweight or "just right." They can be done by women of any age without undue strain. All of them can be done throughout a normal pregnancy with the exception of the overhead reach. All six can be done from a standing position—which should make it extra easy for you to start. They require no special equipment; no special area. All they need is a few minutes of your time every day.

I want to help you get into the habit of exercising regularly. When you become accustomed to doing the Basic Six, you will want to progress with some of the more rigorous exercises. When you discover how *easy* it is to exercise—and see the results for yourself; find out how much better you feel and look—I know you will want to add more and more to your daily routine.

I cannot over-stress the importance of regularity to a successful body-improvement program. It is the repeated action of the muscles, day after day, that brings results. Don't overdo at the beginning. Start with five times for each exercise and add a few more each day. Remember that you are waking up muscles that have been asleep for a long, long time. If you strain them in the beginning, they are going to ache. If you accustom them gradually to the new pull, they will adjust very naturally and you will not suffer any stiffness or soreness.

So start off slowly—even if you feel you could do many more than just five the first day. It is the repetition, day after day, that is going to do the job for you.

Of course, the more you do an exercise, the more it will do for you. But I caution you about overdoing at the beginning because I know that nothing discourages a beginner like an aching back or stiff knees. I want to keep you faithful to your beauty exercises. I would rather see you do the Basic Six every day than to start off trying every exercise in the book in a spurt of enthusiasm—and doing none at all for days afterwards.

Now you're all set to go. You're on your way to a prettier, more youthful and healthier figure.

Debbie's Basic Six

Basic Number One
For the Hips and Thighs

Let's start from the feet up. This exercise works on everything from the ankles to the waist. It's an easy one to begin with and pays big beauty dividends. It slims and firms the hips and thighs, tones the tummy muscles, lifts the rib-cage and gives the body youthful suppleness and grace.

STAND tall and straight, stretching the body to full height. Rest your left hand on a table, the back of a chair, the mantelpiece or kitchen counter—to help you keep your balance. Place your right hand on your waist. 1) Swing the right leg forward as high as you can. 2) Now, swing down again and kick it as far back as you can. Keep the leg and knee straight as you swing; the toes pointed so they will add to the stretch.

Start with five full swings to the right leg. Reverse your position and do five full swings with the left leg. That's enough for the first time. Tomorrow you add another swing or two—and keep adding gradually as you become accustomed to the movement. You should be able to work up to twenty-five full swings with each leg—or more, if you like.

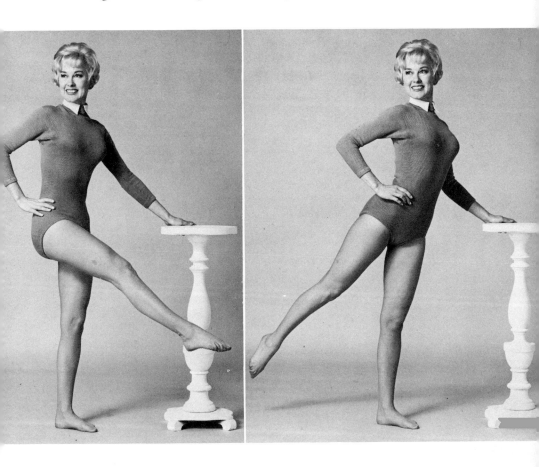

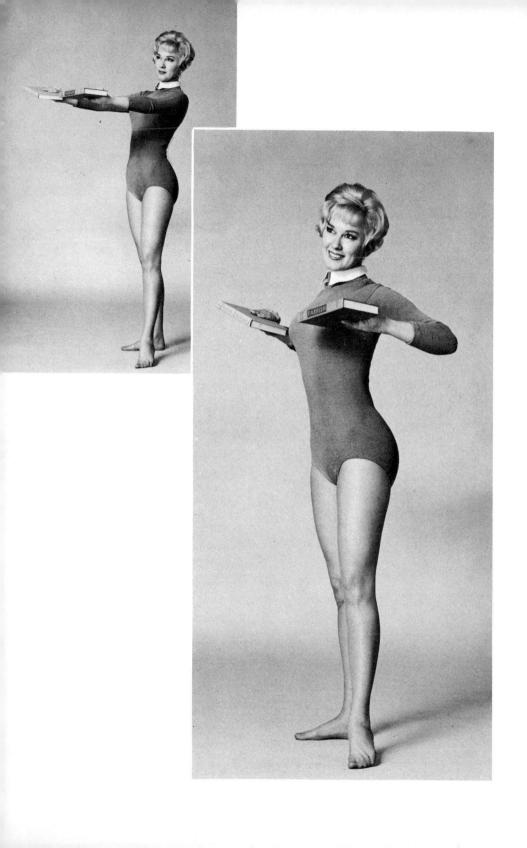

Basic Number Two
For the Bustline and Upper Arms

Let's move on now to the upper torso. This exercise will improve the bustline and the upper arms. When I say "improve"—I mean it is equally good for the underdeveloped bust as for the heavy bosom. It will benefit both thin and heavy arms. Follow the instructions for increasing or decreasing, according to your own figure needs.

For increasing, hold a book in each hand as you do the exercise. Pause after each ten. *For decreasing,* use no weights and repeat without stopping.

In either case, this exercise will lift and firm the bosom. It will keep the upper arm firm and tight and eliminate the flabbiness that so often occurs in this area.

STAND straight and tall. (Any exercise done from a standing position provides an opportunity for improving the posture while reshaping the figure.) 1) Stretch the arms in front of you at chest height. 2) Bring the arms open to the sides with a nice, strong pull. And you should feel that pull in the muscles under the bust and in the arms. Open, close, open, close. Don't forget to hold a book in each hand if you are trying to increase your bust measurements.

Start with this exercise ten times. Add a few counts each day until you reach at least thirty repetitions.

Basic Number Three
For the Arms and Back

This basic exercise trims and firms the arms and back. Many women with otherwise good figures shout their ages with their arms and backs. If you want to look well in the sleeveless and low back fashions—this exercise will do the trick for you. As it firms these two areas, it also pulls in the waistline and lifts the bust.

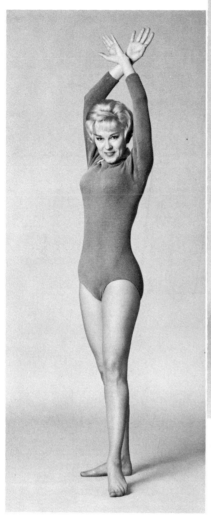
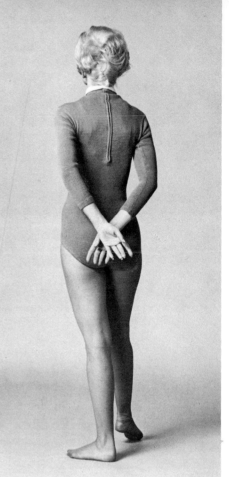

STAND with the feet slightly apart. Drop your arms straight down at the sides of the body. 1) Raise the hands straight out from the sides and up over the head until they cross behind the head. 2) Lower the hands to the sides and cross them again behind the hips. (During pregnancy, do not raise the hands over the head. Lift out to the sides slightly and then cross behind the hips.)

Start with five, increasing daily until you reach twenty-five (or more.)

Basic Number Four
For the Chin and Neckline

The chin and neckline are areas where many women first reveal their ages. This exercise will keep the neckline firm and youthful—and guard against a double chin.

While STANDING, throw the head back. Open the mouth slightly and try to bring the lower lip over the upper lip. Push your chin right up to the ceiling.

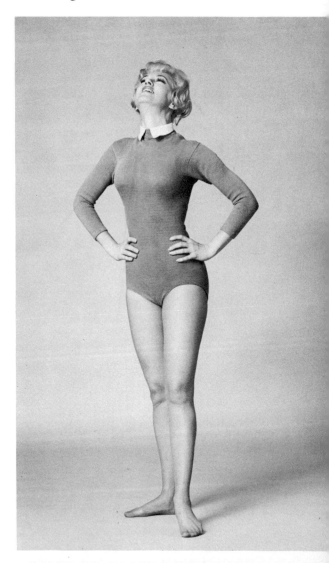

If you have a pronounced double chin, do this exercise whenever you have an opportunity. You may do it while sitting down as well as standing. It is easier to prevent a double chin than to cure one—but remember that persistence pays. Keep at it and you can do a great deal to modify the problem.

Basic Number Five
For the Tummy

This is a simple exercise that can be done by a woman of any age. It tightens and firms the stomach muscles and gives bonus benefits to the hips and thighs, as well.

STAND tall with your hands on your hips. 1) Raise the right knee as high as it will go. 2) Now change and raise the left leg as high as possible. Think of the high-stepping drum majorettes leading a parade as you do this. Put as much action as possible into each movement.

Start with a count of ten. Increase daily until you reach fifty. If you throw your head back as you take your high steps, you will be helping to keep your neckline youthful, too.

Basic Number Six
For the Waistline

The Waist-Bounce is another double-duty exercise. It will help you get—and keep—a slender waistline but it is also very good for relieving tension in the lower back.

From a STANDING position, bend your arms at the elbows and intertwine them. 1) Grasp the right elbow with the left hand—the left elbow with the right hand. 2) Now, bend over at the waist and *bounce* up and down. The more bounce, the more supple and slender your waistline will become.

Start with ten bounces. I know you can do more—easily. But don't overdo on the first day. Keep adding gradually until you can bounce as easily as a ball on a rubber string. Up and down, up and down. Watch that spare tire disappear.

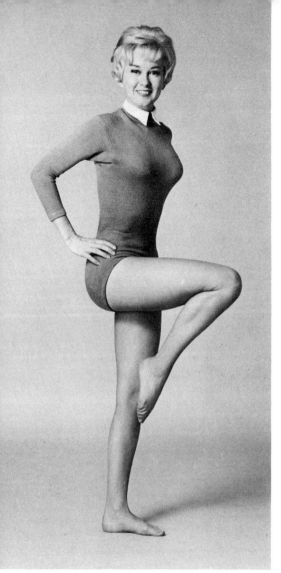

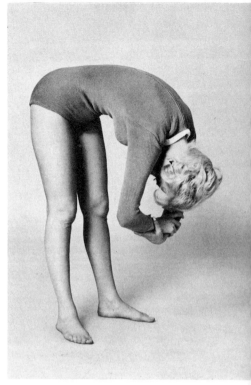

Now that you have mastered the Basic Six—you are ready to go on to the following chapters.

The next step is to decide what your particular figure problems are and select exercises from these special groups to correct them. I enjoy variety in my own exercise routine and always choose a new exercise to add to my daily regimen. Each exercise brings different muscles into play and I find that I can keep my body in top condition by utilizing as many changes of action as possible.

10

Developing
a Beautiful Bustline

Increasing, decreasing,
lifting and firming the bustline

Of all the requests for advice on figure improvement that I receive in the mail, more than one-third concern the bustline. Understandably so, for a lovely bustline is the hallmark of a perfect feminine figure.

Many women believe that this is one area of the body which cannot be changed by exercise or diet. This is not true. I know from personal experience how my own bustline has been developed through exercise. And I have helped many women increase or decrease their busts in both measurement and cup size.

The bosom is affected by weight loss or gain—just as the other parts of the body are. This is very important to remember whether you are trying to increase or decrease. Many women who want to increase their bust measurements are overweight and over-sized in other areas. In order to lose the excess weight they must diet as well as exercise to improve their proportions. Don't become alarmed if the tape measure shows a loss rather than a gain in the total measurement of the bustline. Remember that if you are losing weight, some of it is probably going from across the back as well as in other places. Exercise will build up the bosom itself—which is what we want it to do.

The same theory applies to the woman with a large bust. Dieting will help her go down in her overall bust measurements because she is eliminating the excess fat across the back, but exercise will help her keep the bosom itself full and firm as she wants it to be.

Size is by no means the only problem of the bustline. No bosom, large or small, is attractive if it sags. To keep the bosom well-shaped, high, rounded and firm, you should devote a portion of your daily exercise routine to keeping these muscles well-toned and youthful.

Increasing the Bustline

The principle of weights to increase the pull on the muscles and thereby build them up can be successfully applied to exercises for the bustline. In any bust exercise which leaves the hands free, you should hold a weight in each hand to increase the muscle tension. I use books for this purpose as they are easily obtainable and are of the proper weight.

Most exercises that affect the bustline also affect the muscles of the upper arm. For this reason, I do not recommend the use of heavy dumbbells for they may over-develop the upper arm. No girl wants the arm proportions of a gymnast. The book weights are heavy enough to develop the bosom without pulling too heavily on the arms.

It is important to pause after each ten counts of any bust exercise in which weights are used. You may do as many repeats as you like as long as you remember to stop for a count of five between each series of ten.

In any bust exercise employing weights, do the exercise every other day. The Finger Press, Wrist Push, Elbow Raise and Arm Pushups may be done daily, but the others will give best results if used on alternate days only.

One other suggestion that many have found helpful in stimulating the development of the breasts is the use of alternating hot and cold compresses. It is preferable to follow this procedure while in a reclining position. Wrap a small amount of ice in a clean washcloth and gently massage the breast until the cloth becomes warm. Rinse the cloth with warm water and massage again until the cloth turns cool. Alternate three times with each breast. This routine must be followed daily for a minimum of two months before there will be any noticeable results. After this time, however, you should find there is a definite tendency toward increase in size. This is particularly helpful to the teenage figure which is still in the development stage.

A question that is frequently asked by the women who write to me is whether anything can be done to balance the size of the bosom. In many cases, one breast tends to be smaller than the other. This situation is entirely natural and is no cause for alarm. The only suggestion I can offer in correcting this problem is to do extra exercises for increasing using only the arm which is on the side of the smaller breast. You might also try using a heavier book weight with that arm when doing the Flys and Pull-Overs.

Increasing the bustline calls for patience. The exercises do not bring immediate results. They must be repeated regularly for a period of several months before an increase occurs. It will encourage you to know, however, that these exercises will start to lift and firm the bust right from the start. And any bosom, however small, is more attractive when it is higher and more firm. Content yourself with the knowledge that you *are* improving your bustline even though the tape measure may not show an increase in size immediately.

Decreasing the Bustline

An extremely heavy bust is usually an indication of a general overweight problem. For exercises to be fully effective in reducing the size of the bust, they should be done in accompaniment to a reducing diet. As you shed the excess fat by dieting, it will be easier to decrease the bust measurements by exercise.

Bust exercises are extremely important for the dieter as they will prevent sagging and keep the bosom well-shaped and firm as you lose weight. When exercising for a decrease in bust measurements, use no weights. Repeat each exercise for at least twenty times without stopping and do them regularly every day.

Exercises for the Bustline

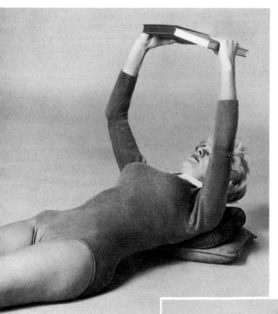

The Flys

Starting Position: LIE DOWN on your back. Place a pillow under the shoulders. 1) Raise the arms above the chest as though you were holding a barrel. 2) Open the curved arms as widely as possible, pulling them way back. 3) Return arms to front of chest. TO INCREASE: Hold a book in each hand and repeat ten times. Rest through a count of five. Repeat another ten times. You may do as many as you like as long as you pause between each ten Flys. TO DECREASE: Do the Flys without book weights and repeat twenty times (or more) without stopping.

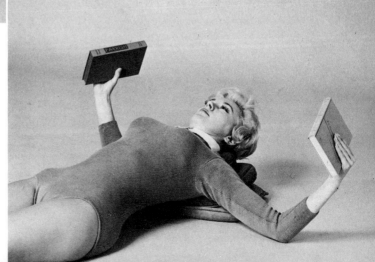

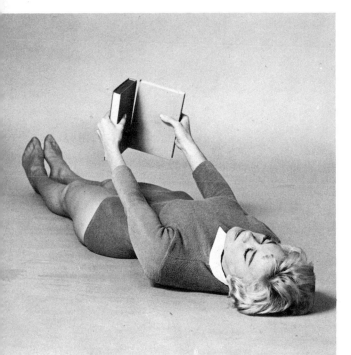

Circle Flys

Starting Position: LIE DOWN on your back (without pillow support). Extend arms to full length downward, hands touching. 1) Bending the elbows, raise the hands up to the sides of the head, as though you were drawing an arc. 2) Return hands downward in same cycle. TO INCREASE: Hold a book in each hand during exercise. Repeat ten times. Rest through a count of five. Repeat. Rest. TO DECREASE: Do Circle Flys without book weights and repeat twenty times (or more) without stopping.

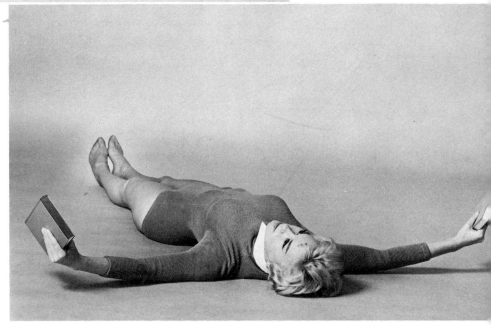

Pull-Overs
(Increasing Only)

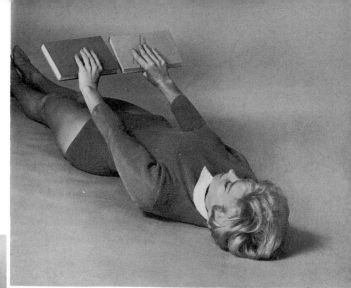

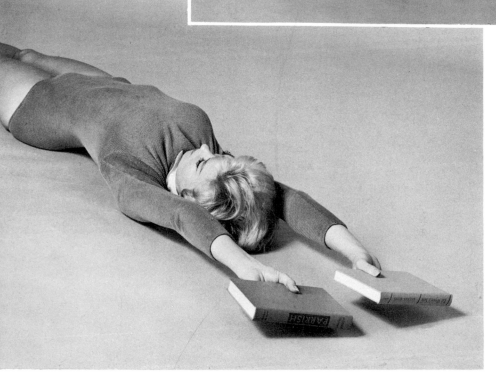

Starting Position: LIE DOWN on your back. Hold a book in each hand. 1) Extend arms straight out toward knees. 2) Raise the books over the head, reaching as far back as possible until they touch the floor behind the head. 3) Return to starting position.

The arms must be kept straight at all times. Repeat ten times, rest through a count of five. Repeat as often as you like, resting between each ten Pull-Overs.

Debbie's Daily Double

This one is a great favorite of mine. It combines the Flys and the Pull-Overs. LIE DOWN on the floor and hold the arms above the chest in the barrel position described in The Flys. Open the arms out to the sides of the body as far as they will go. Return. Now raise the arms above the head until they touch the floor behind the head as in Pull-Overs. Return. Alternate and repeat. Remember the rules for increasing and decreasing. TO INCREASE: Hold a book in each hand. Do ten, rest, repeat. TO DECREASE: Use no book weights and repeat twenty times or more without stopping.

For variety, try these first four exercises from a standing position. They are equally effective done this way. As long as you feel the pull through the bustline, you know you are getting results.

Finger Press

This is an easy exercise that can be done from a seated or standing position. It firms and lifts the bust and tightens the upper arm. It is good for you whether you are trying to increase or decrease. 1) Bend the elbows at chest level. 2) With the palms outstretched, let the fingers of one hand touch those of the other. 3) PRESS the fingers together as hard as you can. You will feel the pull as you press. Repeat twenty times or more.

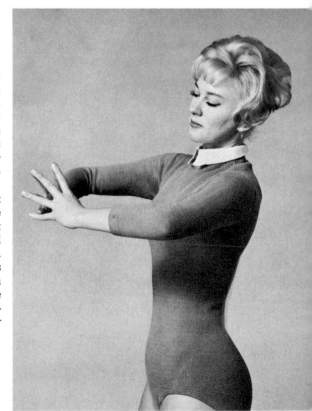

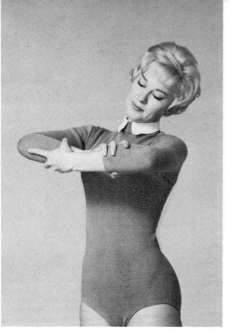

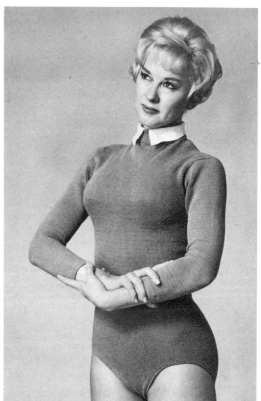

Wrist Push

(Seated or standing position.) 1)
Bend the elbows at chest level.
Hold the left wrist with the right
hand; the right wrist with the left
hand. 2) PUSH the hands vigorously toward the elbows. Here
again, you will feel the action on
the bust muscles as you push.
Twenty times or more.

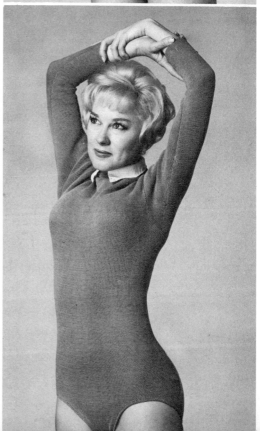

Elbow Raise

Starting Position: STAND with
arms crossed at chest level. Hold
the right elbow with the left hand;
the left elbow with the right hand.
1) Raise the elbows over the head,
reaching as far back as you can. It's
the pull back that brings results.
2) Return arms to chest level. Repeat twenty times or more.

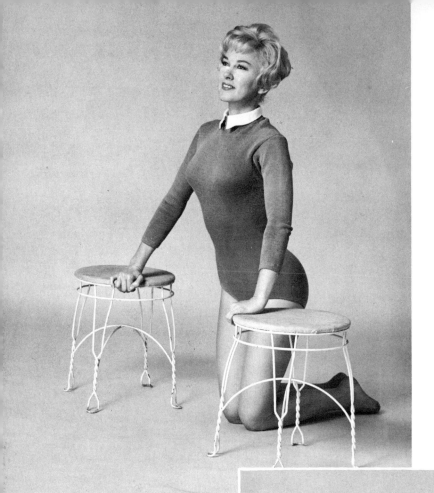

Arm Pushups

For this exercise, you will need two chairs or small stools. Place the chairs about two feet apart. Starting position: KNEEL on the floor and place one hand on each chair seat. 1) Keeping your weight on your arms, raise the chest until the arms are straight. 2) Lower the chest, bending the elbows as you go down.

Start slowly with this exercise. Five is the most you should do for the first few times. Gradually increase until you reach a total of fifteen or twenty arm pushups.

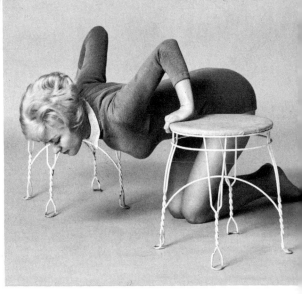

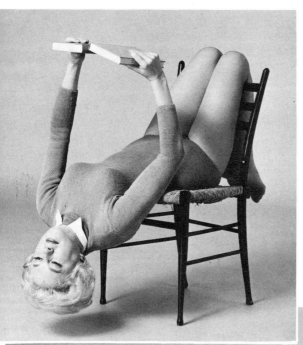

Chair Flys

This requires a straight back chair. Starting Position: Rest the hips on the chair seat and hook the knees over the back of the chair. Drop the head down to the floor. 1) Bring the arms up to chest level and curve them as though you were holding a barrel. 2) Pull the arms open to the sides as far as you can. 3) Return arms to chest level. TO IN-CREASE: Hold a book in each hand and rest briefly after each ten. TO DE-CREASE: Use no book weights and repeat twenty times or more without stop-ping.

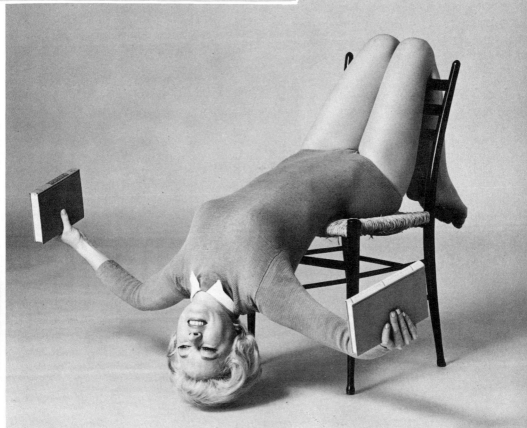

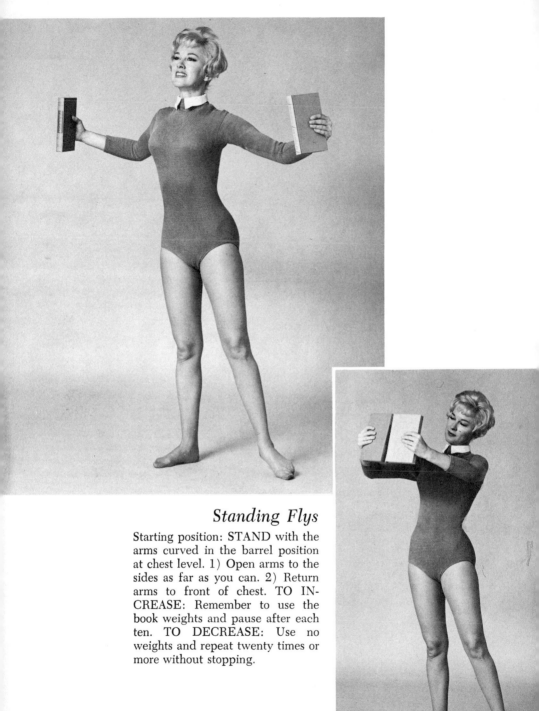

Standing Flys

Starting position: STAND with the arms curved in the barrel position at chest level. 1) Open arms to the sides as far as you can. 2) Return arms to front of chest. TO IN-CREASE: Remember to use the book weights and pause after each ten. TO DECREASE: Use no weights and repeat twenty times or more without stopping.

11

Slimming, Shaping and Firming the Hips and Thighs

I group the hips and thighs together in this chapter because it is practically impossible to separate these two areas in exercises. The hip and upper thigh are affected by the same exercises and for the most part, any exercise that helps the thighs, helps the hips—and vice versa.

Dieting will reduce the bulk of a padded hip or heavy thigh —but only exercise will keep these areas firm and shapely. Even girls with well-proportioned lower torsos find themselves with problems when the bathing suit season arrives. Too much winter sitting, the wearing of girdles and the absence of regular exercising create an extra bulge in the hips and flabbiness through the thighs.

Constant leg-crossing will also tend to produce flabbiness . . . particularly in the inner thigh. If you sit at a desk a great deal, get in the habit of sitting well back in your chair with the knees together and the feet resting squarely on the floor. Practice getting up and down from your chair without supporting yourself with your hands. This action pulls and strengthens the thigh muscles and keeps them firm.

Walking and stair-climbing are basic hip and thigh improvement exercises. Bicycling is the best sports activity there is for slimming and firming hips and thighs. Golf and tennis are also excellent and provide an easy way to have fun while you are improving your figure.

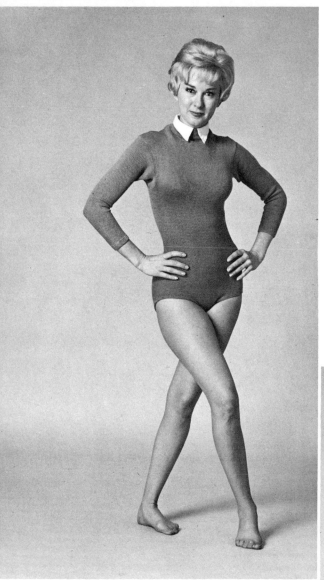

Debbie's Walker

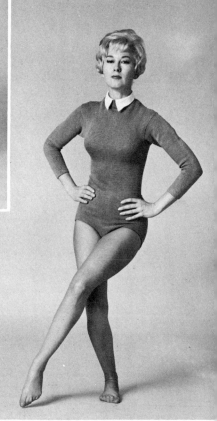

This exercise is good for any type of hip and thigh problem. It firms and slims, shapes and trims.

Starting position: STAND with your hands on your hips. 1) Cross the right leg over the left knee and step forward with a deep knee bend. 2) Cross the left leg over the right knee and step forward again with another deep knee bend. You will feel the pull through the thighs as you walk. Don't overdo this one at the beginning but add a few more steps each day as the muscles become accustomed to the pull.

The Squats

The Squats are good for everyone. Vary the way you do them according to your figure needs. They are also excellent preparation for active sports. They will take the "kinks" out of the golfer, skier, tennis player, horsewoman and swimmer. The Squats are beneficial during pregnancy, too, for they limber up the lower torso and help prepare for delivery, and also keep the hips and thighs firm.

Squats for Reducing

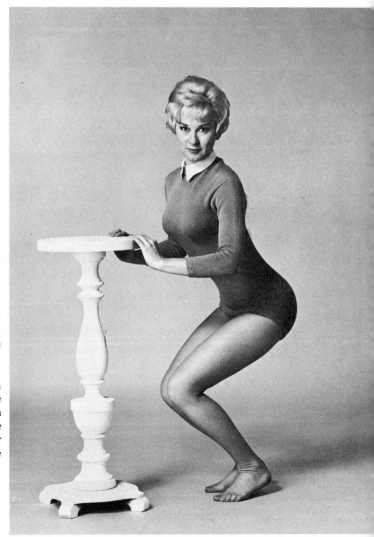

Starting position: STAND with both hands touching the back of a chair, a table, kitchen counter or other similar support. 1) Slowly lower the body from a standing position to a squatting position. The knees bend as you go down but the back remains straight. 2) Slowly, rise again. As you will find when you practice this, the slower the up and down motion, the deeper the pull. And the deeper the pull, the better the results.

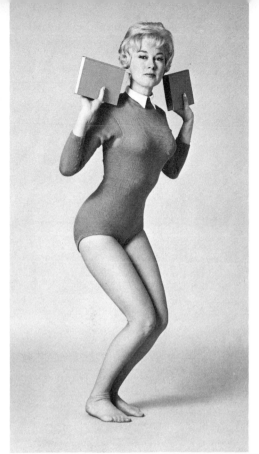

Squats for Increasing

Do the squats as described above but instead of holding on to a chair or other support, hold a book at shoulder height (one in each hand) as you go up and down. This will challenge your balancing powers but after a little practice you will become more sure-footed.

Sitting Scissors Kicks

This requires a straight chair. Starting position: SIT UP with your back settled firmly against the back of the chair. Fold your arms together in back of the chair. Stretch your legs straight out in front of you with toes pointed forward. 1) Raise both legs off the floor and kick rapidly up and down, up and down, as fast as you can go. Keep the knees stiff and the legs as high as you can.

This may wear you out a little at first, but keep it up every day and you will find that your legs can go higher each time and the speed of your kicks will increase. (P.S. to office workers: this is a great cure for the secretarial spread!)

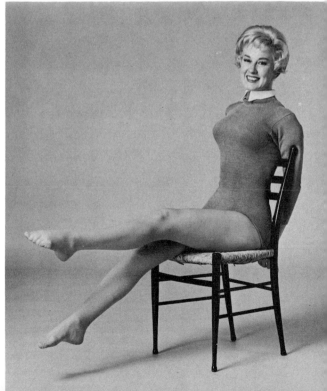

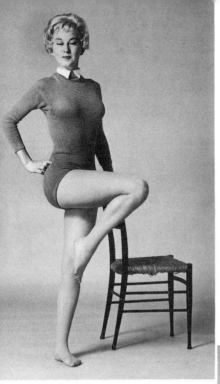

The Knee Swing

Here again, we need a chair. This exercise works on the bulging hip and the flabby thigh, but it is also good for building up in these areas. That's the magic of exercise. So often what is good for reducing works just as well for building up. It is all a matter of putting the muscles into proper working order and firming the skin tissues.

Starting position: STAND and hold on to the back of a chair with your left hand. Right hand should be on the hip. 1) Bring the right knee up into the tummy. 2) Swing the knee around to the left side. 3) Swing the knee around to the right side. Back and forth as far as you can to each side. Do ten swings with the right knee. Reverse position and do ten swings with the left knee.

Always begin a new exercise with a minimum number of counts. Ten to each leg is enough for the first day. Add a few more counts each day as you go along and work up to as many as you have time and energy for. Remember, the more you do, the more you accomplish.

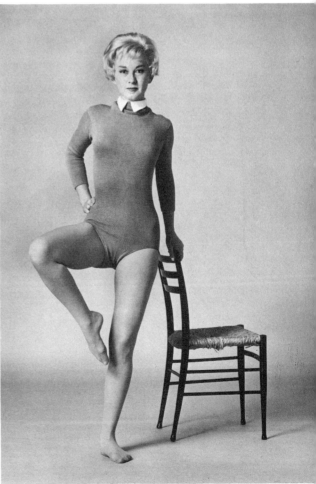

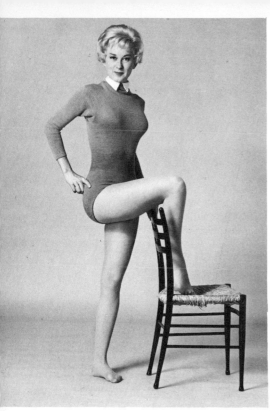

The Swing-Over

The Swing-Over requires a chair, too. Starting position: Stand sidewards behind the chair and hold on to the chair back with your left hand. 1) Bring the right leg up and over the back of the chair until your foot touches the seat. 2) Bring the leg down again and 3) stretch it out in back of the left leg. Repeat for ten swings with the right leg. Reverse positions and repeat for ten swings with the left leg. That's enough for the first day. Add a few swings each time until you are doing a total of at least fifty.

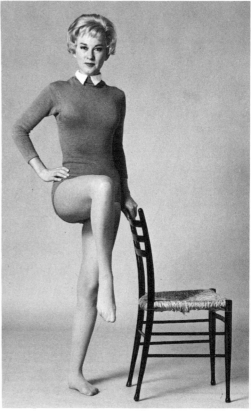

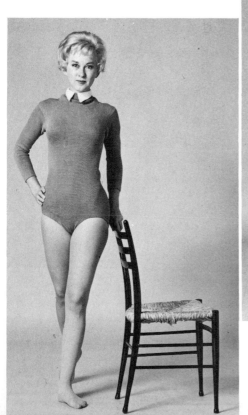

Lunges (Increasing Only)

This is the best exercise I know for building up the thighs into more attractive contours. Starting position: STAND straight with your hands at your waist. 1) Step forward with the right foot. 2) Bend the right knee deeply down as far as you can, shifting all the weight onto the forward leg. 3) Return right leg to starting position. 4) Step forward with left leg and repeat the action, putting all your weight on the left leg. Alternate, doing a total of five lunges with each leg, adding a few each day until you reach a total of thirty or more.

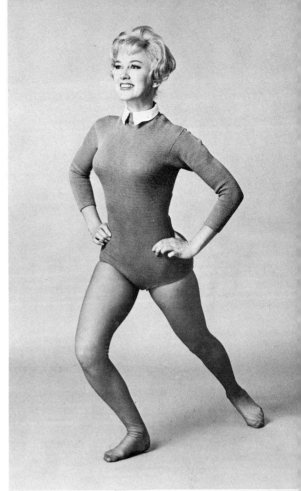

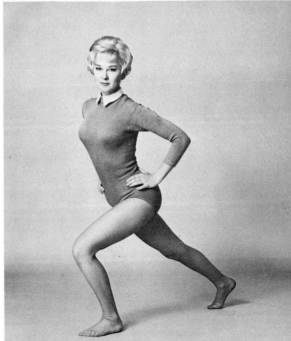

The Bicycle

This is an old-timer, but it is still one of the best exercises ever devised for slimming the hips and thighs. Starting position: LIE DOWN on your back with a pillow under your hips. 1) Raise hips and legs off the floor at right angles to the upper part of the body. 2) With strong, stretching movements, bicycle as though you were out to win a race! You will want to support your hips with your hands for balance. Ride this homemade bicycle every day if you want to whittle away that extra fat on your hips and thighs.

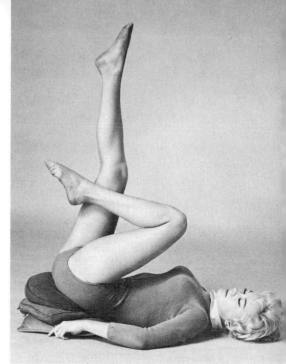

The Bounce

Here's one that will bounce away the bulges. This is particularly good for the heavy, firm upper thigh that needs real breaking down in order to reduce (and it's a lot less expensive than reducing machines and massages.)

Starting position: LIE DOWN on the floor on your right side. Stretch the body out to full length. Put your left hand on the floor in front of your waist; your right hand on the floor above your head. 1) Raise the body up and down from the floor. Give your hips a good bounce against the floor as you come down. Start with ten good bounces on the right side; alternate to ten bounces on the left side. That's enough for the first time, but keep increasing the number each day.

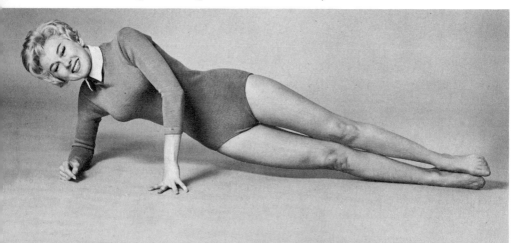

Leg-Overs

Time to get down on the floor, now. Many of the exercises which slice away the hip pads and thigh bulges are done from a prone position. The floor serves as a hard surface against which you can literally roll or bounce away the fat. Many women are cursed with an ugly bulge where the thigh joins the hip. This type of bulge ruins the body line in a bathing suit, slacks or sheath skirts. This exercise can make that bulge melt away if you keep at it regularly.

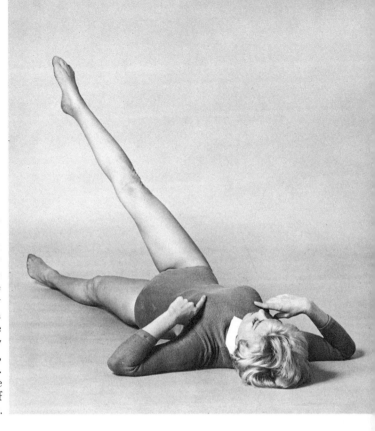

Starting position: LIE DOWN on your back with your hands at your chest. 1) Raise the right leg straight up into the air. 2) Cross the leg over the body until it touches the floor on the left side. 3) Return leg to starting position. 4) Repeat with left leg, crossing over to floor on right side. Alternate, starting with a total of ten and working up gradually to at least thirty. (More if you're serious about eliminating that bulge.)

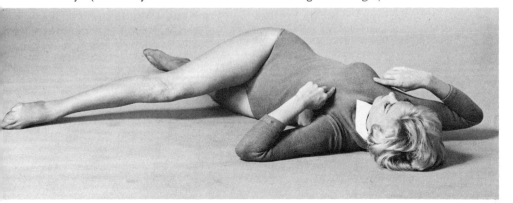

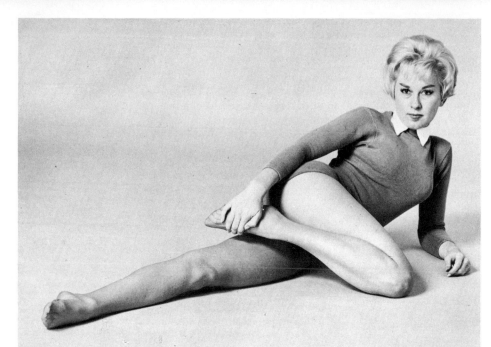

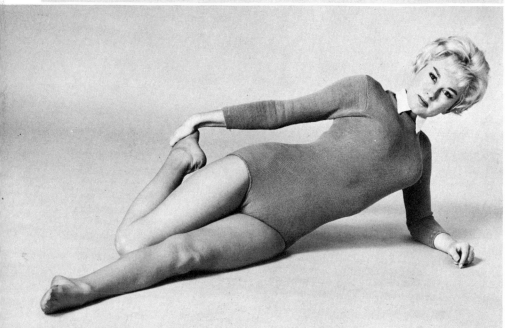

Knees-Over

This is another double-duty exercise for the hips and thighs. And it slims the tummy, too. Starting position: LIE ON THE LEFT SIDE, stretched to full length. 1) Grasp the right foot with the right hand. 2) Bring the right knee forward and 3) touch the floor in front of the body. 4) Swing the knee over and touch the floor in back of the body. Repeat ten times with the right knee. Reverse position and do ten Knee-Overs with the left knee. Work up to as many counts as you can, always alternating after each ten.

Foot-Overs

Starting position: LIE DOWN on your back. Raise the body off the floor, supporting the weight with your heels and hands. 1) Bend the right knee and 2) touch the floor on the left side with the right foot. 3) Bring knee back to the center of the body and 4) return right leg to floor. Alternate from right to left leg, starting with a total of ten and adding a few more counts each day.

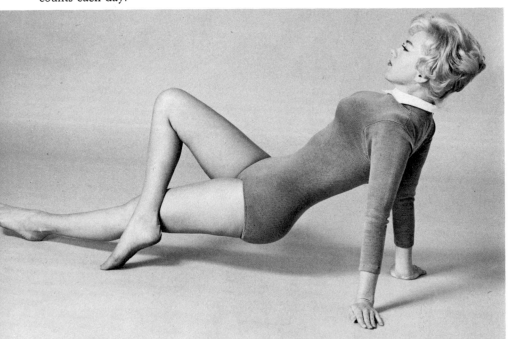

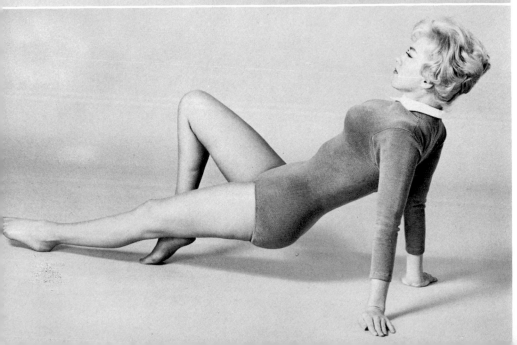

Knee Press

This exercise is so simple and it is sheer magic for the thighs. You can do this exercise at your office desk or while sitting at the breakfast table and no one will be the wiser. It is just as effective with shoes on as without them. I recommend this for everyone, slim and heavy, too solid or too flabby. It hits directly at the inner thigh muscles. You can feel the muscles tense and relax as you do it.

Starting position: SITTING DOWN with both feet on the floor. 1) Turn the toes outward, keeping a distance of about eighteen inches between the feet. 2) Bring the knees together and 3) press the knees firmly into each other. Press, relax, press, relax. Keep this up and your upper legs will become firm and youthfully shaped.

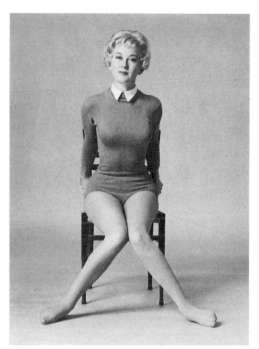

Leg Stretch

This is another exercise you can do while seated. It works on the thighs but gives you a beauty bonus for it also firms the stomach muscles. Starting position: SIT on the edge of your chair with legs together and pulled slightly under the chair. 1) Lift the legs forward and extend them straight out. 2) Hold legs in this position briefly and 3) return feet to floor. Do this exercise slowly because it is holding the legs at tension that tenses and pulls the muscles. If you merely swing the legs up and down, you will not accomplish the purpose. You may also do this exercise with just one leg at a time.

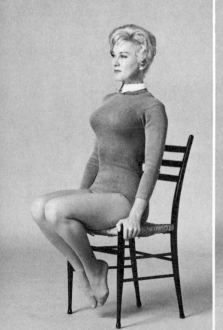

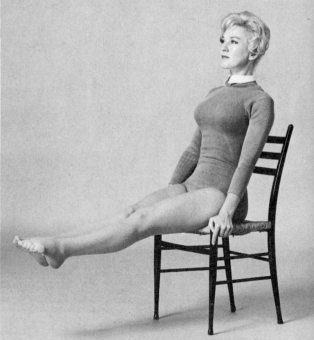

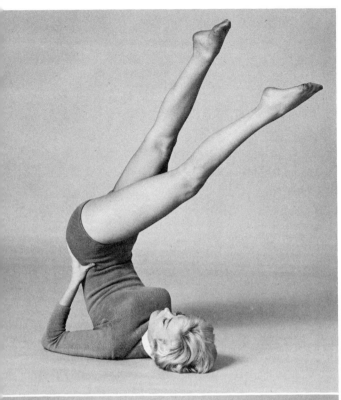

Scissor Kicks

These may be done two days. I always do a group of cross-kicks, then a group of forward kicks, alternating after each twenty or so. Starting position: LIE DOWN on your back. You may use a pillow under the hips, if you wish. Raise the hips and legs straight up in the air at right angles to the body. 1) Swing the legs to opposite sides of the body, crossing them in the air. 2) Swing the legs back and forth, scissor style. I caution you not to overdo these at the beginning. But try to work up to a good number of them in time as they are so beneficial for the hips and thighs. They shape, trim, curve and firm.

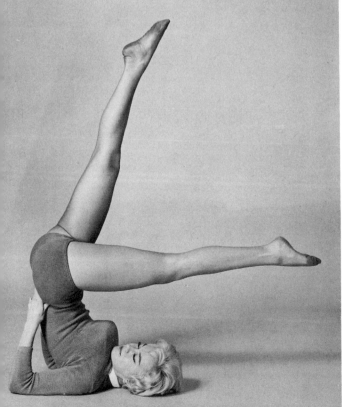

Giant Steps (For Building Up)

TO INCREASE the curves on the hips and thighs, do this one. Starting position: GET DOWN ON THE FLOOR on the hands and feet. Keep the hips straight and 1) Take a forward step with the right leg. 2) Return the right leg to position and 3) Take a forward step with the left leg. This should be done rapidly at a running speed even though the body remains in one place. Start with a few and work up to as many as you like.

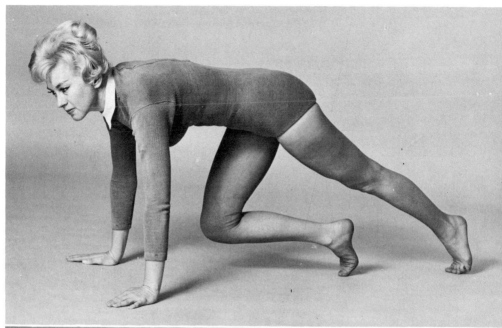

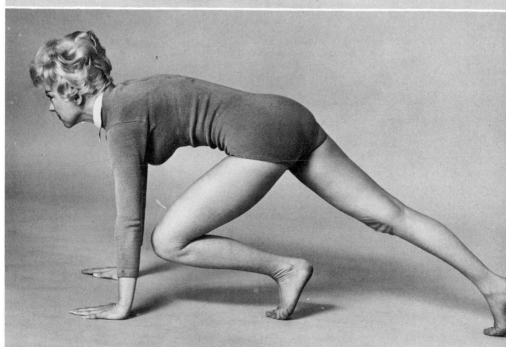

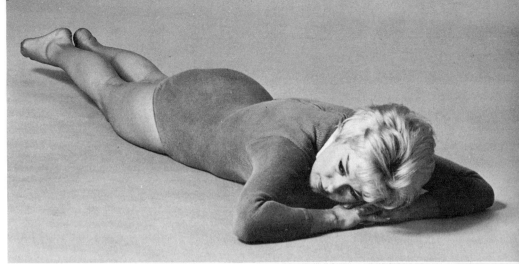

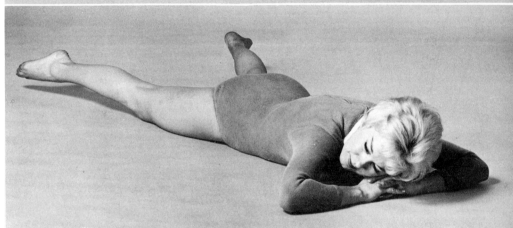

Floor-Swings

Starting position: LIE DOWN on the tummy, legs outstretched. 1) Raise the legs slightly off the floor. 2) Swing the legs open. 3) Close legs again —keeping them off the floor.

This exercise is terrific for the hips and thighs and also pulls on the tummy muscles as you will discover when you do it.
(The same exercise can be done while lying on the back.)

Firming the Inner Thighs

So many women write to me complaining about flabbiness on their inner thighs. Even a well-proportioned leg loses its attractiveness if the skin is loose and crêpe-like. To keep the inner thigh firm and youthful, do this exercise regularly. You will remember that I included this exercise as one of the Basic Six. It pays big beauty dividends for it helps to shape the entire lower torso to more graceful proportions.

Leg Swings

Starting position: STAND sideways holding on to the back of a chair or a table. 1) Swing the outside leg forward and 2) swing back as far as you can go. Reverse position after ten full swings and repeat with the other leg.

You may vary this by alternating with a *side-to-side* swing but be careful not to swing the leg straight out and high at the outside as this tends to produce a crevice between the thigh and hip that is unsightly. You should feel a definite pull on the inner thigh as you swing forward and backward.

Leg Circles

This exercise should be done in accompaniment with Leg Swings to firm the inner thighs.

Starting position: STAND, holding on to the back of a chair or table, with the weight resting on the left foot. 1) Extend the right foot forward and out, with the toe pointed. 2) With the extended toe, draw circles in the air. The wider the circles, the greater the pull. Repeat for ten times and reverse, doing the same movement with the other leg. Alternate and repeat as long as you like.

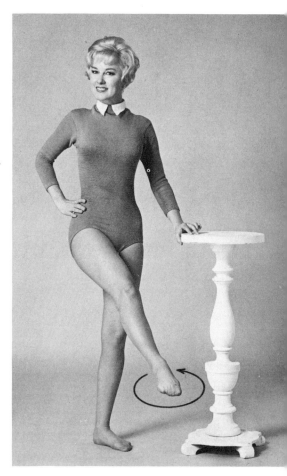

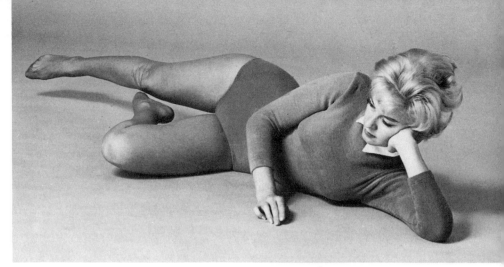

Side Bicycles

This exercise works directly on the outer thighs. The hips and the inner thighs benefit as well, but it is especially helpful for reducing the outer thighs.

Starting position: LIE DOWN on your side with legs outstretched. 1) Bring the knees up alternately and push the leg straight again just as though you were riding a bicycle. This exercise pushes away at the bulges. Be sure to alternate so that each side gets equal action.

Reducing the Outer Thighs

Side Bounce

This is the same as The Bounce. I repeat it because it is especially good for reducing the outer thighs. Do it in combination with Side Bicycles.

Starting position: LIE DOWN on your side with the lower arm stretched out above the head and the outer arm on the floor at the front of the waist. 1) *Bounce* good and hard on the outside of the thighs. Reverse sides, giving each a thorough workout.

Shaping the Buttocks

Rounding and firming the buttocks is another figure problem about which women frequently ask. Often the buttocks soften with age and drop down, increasing the girth of the hips. Here the problem is actually one of re-shaping the buttocks— rather than of reducing the hips. Here are two exercises that will prove rewarding if this has happened to you.

Back Kicks (Standing)

Starting position: STAND facing the back of a chair and holding it with both hands. 1) With the knees straight, kick one leg backwards as far as it will go, extending the toes as you kick. 2) Repeat with other leg. Alternate after each ten kicks.

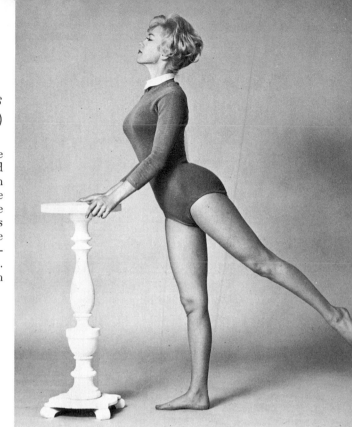

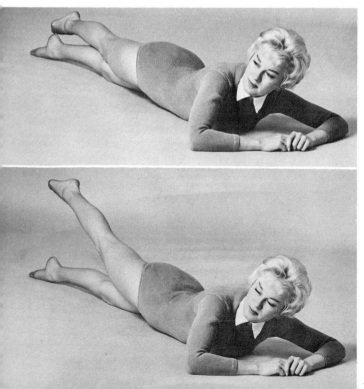

Back Kicks (Lying Down)

Starting position: LIE DOWN on the tummy. 1) Cross one leg slightly over the other and 2) Kick back as high as possible. Kick with one leg ten times. Alternate to other leg for ten kicks. Start with ten for each leg and gradually work up to more, alternating after each ten.

12

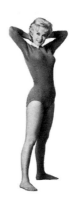

The
Waistliners

Getting rid of
the "spare tire"

Just about everyone seems to be fighting the battle of the bulge these days. Men have the problem as much as women. With most people, the waistline is the spot where the first extra pound settles. How many times have you had to loosen your belt an extra notch when leaving the dinner table?

Many women with otherwise excellent figures find themselves acquiring that little extra roll of fat around the waistline that has been dubbed a "spare tire." A girdle only seems to accentuate the problem for it pushes the fat up and over the midriff.

A slim, supple waistline is an asset for every woman. Doctors have as much as said that you can measure your life expectancy with your waistline. To be healthier as well as more attractive, you should strive for a streamlined middle. We think of a lean midriff as a characteristic of youth—but actually any

woman can retain this asset throughout her lifetime if she will
do a few waistline exercises daily.

All waistline exercises are variations of the bends. When the
body bends or twists across the waist, the muscles in the mid-
section are pulled and tightened. The waistline can be made
to stretch out like a rubber band and contract to firm, supple
trimness. The more elasticity you can achieve in your waistline movements, the more quickly your bulges will disappear.

Many women complain that they cannot touch their toes
when they try waist bends. If you are thick waisted, you
undoubtedly have trouble getting down there in the beginning. But as you do these exercises regularly, you will be
proud to discover that it becomes easier each day. Remember
the example of the rubber band: Bend and stretch as though
you were pulling open a rubber band. With practice, your
waist will respond to this movement and you will be on your
way to a slim, youthful midriff.

Incidentally, one of the most valuable exercises anyone with
a bulgy mid-section can practice is the vigorous shaking of
the head "NO" when the second helpings are passed. Diet and
exercise go together to create a slender waistline.

The Waist Bounce

(This is one of the Basic Six as you will recall.) *Starting
position:* STAND with your feet a comfortable distance apart.
Intertwine your arms, grasping the right elbow with the left
hand, the left elbow with the right hand. 1) Bend over at the
waist and 2) Bounce up and down. Let the upper torso hang
loosely from the waist and go up and down, pulling down on
the waist as you go. Start with ten times, adding a few each
day. This exercise is full of dividends, for as you streamline
your waist, you are pulling and firming the leg muscles and
tightening the abdomen.

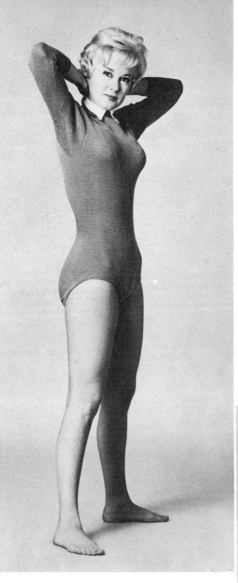

The Zig-Zag

Starting position: STAND with legs apart. Clasp your hands behind your neck. 1) Bend over at the waist and 2) Try to touch your left knee with your right elbow. 3) Return to standing position and bend again, touching the right knee with the left elbow.

You may not be able to reach the knees the first few times, but as your body adjusts to the stretch, you will find yourself able to do so quite easily.

Alternate, right and left, starting with a few and working up to twenty-five or more daily. There's a beauty bonus here, too. This exercise firms the upper arms and the legs as it whittles the waist.

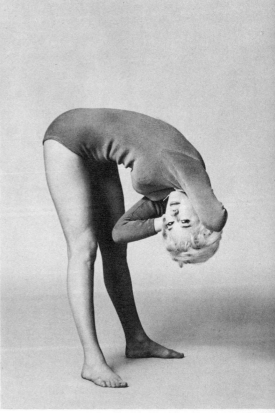

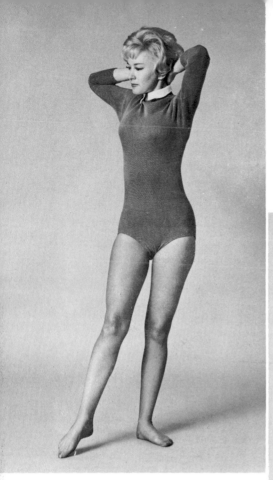

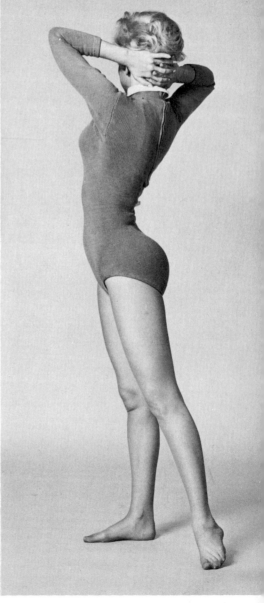

The Twist

This is a variation of the Zig-Zag. In the same starting position: STANDING, with the legs apart, hands clasped behind the neck, 1) Turn the upper half of the body as far to the left as you can go. 2) Turn the body as far to the right as you can go. Practice this one repeatedly and you will find that you are able to swivel the upper torso around to the point where you are almost facing backwards, though your feet remain firmly facing forward. (More extra benefits here for the upper arms and the bustline.)

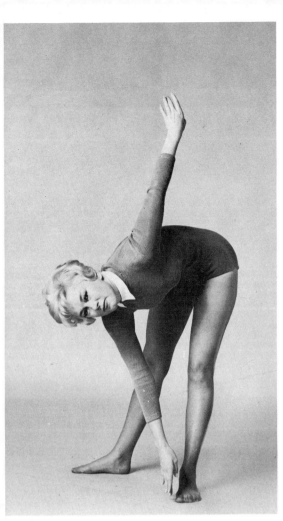

The Toe Touch

Starting position: STAND tall with your hands extended outwards at the sides of your body. 1) Bend over at the waist. 2) Touch the right hand to the left toes. 3) Straighten up and bend again and 4) *repeat on the same side*. Do ten on each side before reversing.

The Floor Touch

Starting position: STAND tall with the feet apart. Place the hands at the waist. 1) Twist the upper torso around to the right. 2) Bend and 3) Touch the floor on the outside of the right foot with *both* hands. 4) Straighten and return hands to the waistline. Reverse, touching floor on outside of the left foot with both hands. Straighten, twist, bend, touch. Alternate. Straighten, twist, bend, touch.

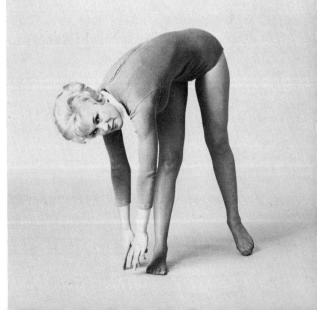

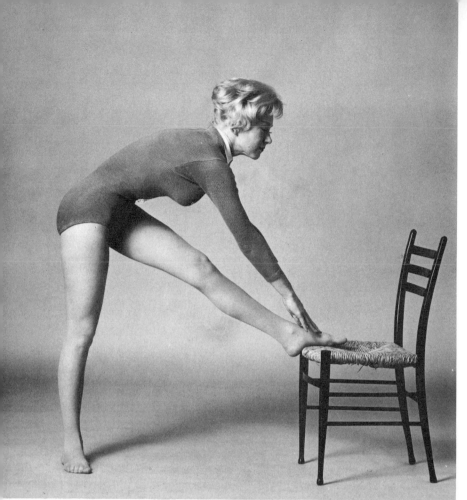

The Chair-Reach

You will need a straight chair for this one.

Starting position: STAND next to the chair and place the right foot on the chair seat. 1) Bend from the waist and 2) Touch the right foot with both hands. 3) Straighten and 4) Touch the left foot (on the floor) with both hands. Alternate. This is excellent for the thighs and calves, as well as the waist.

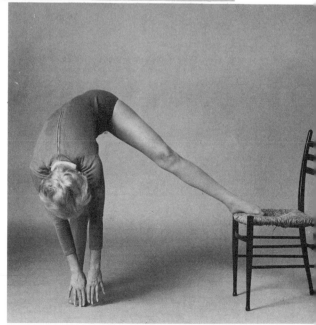

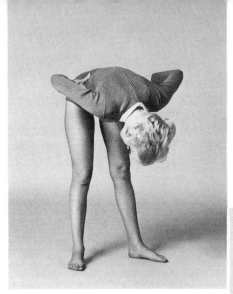

Waist Circles

Starting position: STAND tall with hands at waist. 1) Bend forward from the waist and 2) with the entire top of the body, make big circles. Bend in each direction as far as you can go—forward, side, back, side, forward, etc. Remember it is the pull that slims your waistline. To get full value out of this exercise, you should feel the stretch as you move.

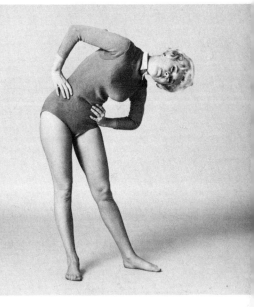

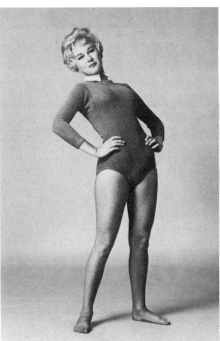

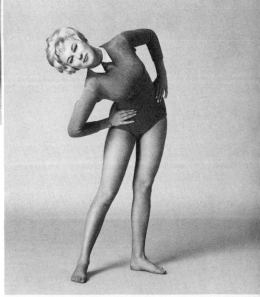

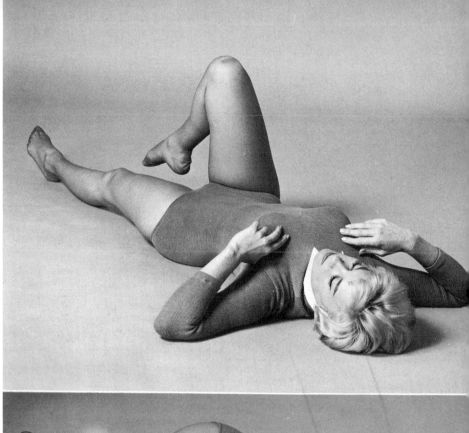

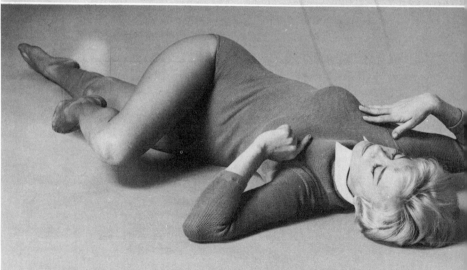

Leg-Overs

What is good for the hips is also good for the waist. This exercise was listed in the chapter dealing with hips and thighs. I repeat it now because it is excellent for the waist, too.

Starting position: LIE DOWN on your back, legs straight out. 1) Bring the right knee up into the tummy. 2) Twist to the left and 3) Bring the right knee to the floor on the left side. Return to starting position and do the same movement with the left knee. Be sure to keep your shoulders flat on the floor as you twist to get the maximum pull through the waist.

Seated Toe-Touch

Starting position: SIT ON THE FLOOR and extend your arms straight out at the sides at shoulder level. The feet should be about eighteen inches apart. 1) Swing the right arm downward and 2) Touch the left toes with your right hand. AT THE SAME TIME, let your left arm swing around to the back. Alternate, touching the right toes with the left hand and swing the right arm to the back. Work up to a rhythmical swinging motion. If you can't touch the toes at the beginning, it only proves how much you need this waist slimming exercise. After a few tries, it will become easier.

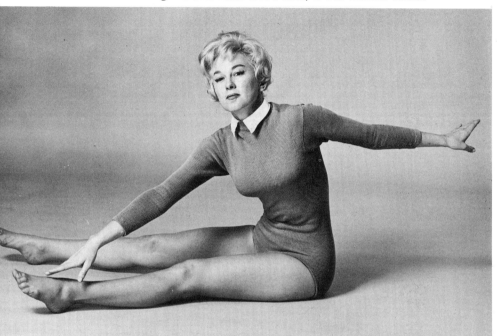

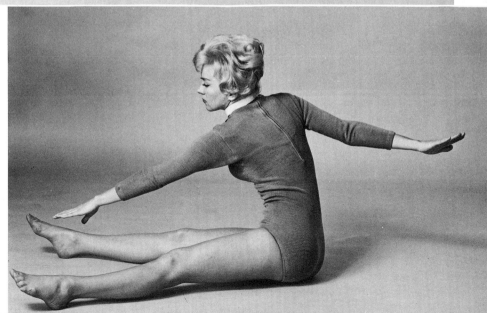

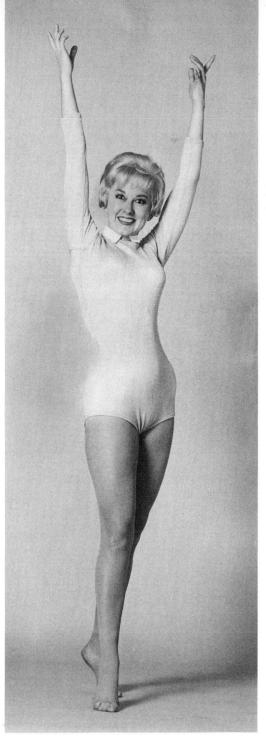

Easy Does It

This is so simple, you may not believe that it can be counted as an exercise. But it is the most important waist-reducer of all.

STAND straight and tall, pull in your tummy and lift the rib-cage. Maintaining this posture when you stand and walk keeps the muscles taut. Often that extra roll at the waistline is the result of poor posture. When you slump, the skin in the mid-section is pushed together, forming a bulge. You can take an inch off your waistline by merely pulling yourself up to full height and raising the rib-cage. This posture exercise is equally important for the stomach and it teaches the tummy muscles to be firm and tight at all times.

13

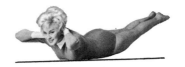

Tightening and
Reducing the Tummy

What shape is your tummy in? I mean when you take your girdle off! Most women are so dependent upon corsetry to hold in their figures, they forget that the stomach was intended to be flat and firm with no help from foundation garments. The shock sets in when they climb into a bathing suit and discover their tummies as they actually are. A flat, firm abdomen is the direct result of muscle control. Of course, overweight women are carrying extra layers of fat in this area and they must diet to get rid of the excess. But many women with slim figures have flabby tummies because they have neglected to exercise these important muscles. The reason many girls have a difficult time getting their figures back after having babies is that their stomach muscles have never been disciplined. If they had been, they would snap back into shape quickly and easily after childbirth.

The number one rule for acquiring a flat tummy is a posture rule. Keep the stomach muscles tensed and pulled in *at all times*—when sitting, standing or walking. Flexing these muscles is a form of exercising them. If you have been guilty of poor posture, you will have to work hard on reminding yourself to pull in the stomach. Start with a daily routine of tensing-relaxing, tensing-relaxing these muscles. The more conscious you are of your tummy, the more you are going to remember to do something about it. Never let a thought about your figure pass through your mind without automatically pulling in the abdomen.

And no cheating! I know all too many women who will maintain graceful posture when they are in company, but in the privacy of their own homes will let their posture collapse. Good posture is a habit. Once acquired, it is a lifetime asset. Good posture improves the appearance of any figure, regardless of size and weight.

Here are some exercises especially designed to reduce a heavy stomach and to tighten, firm and flatten all tummies.

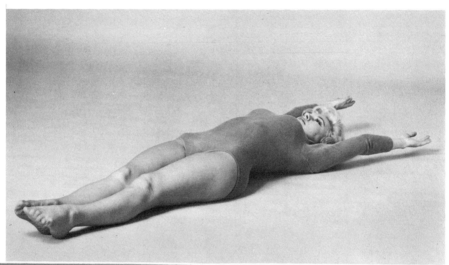

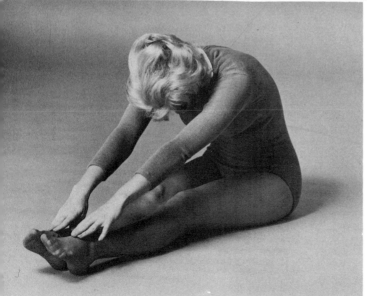

Sit-Ups

Starting position: LIE DOWN on your back with arms outstretched to full length above your head. 1) Raise the body to sitting position. 2) Pull the arms up and forward and touch the toes. Return to starting position. Repeat. You should feel the pull on your stomach muscles as you go up and down.

Leg-Raise

Starting position: LIE DOWN on your back with the hands under the hips. 1) Raise the right leg up off the floor until it is perpendicular to the body. 2) Lower leg to the floor. 3) Now raise the left leg in the same manner and lower. Alternate with the right and left legs as many times as you can, starting with ten raises and increasing daily.

You may vary this one by raising both legs at one time.

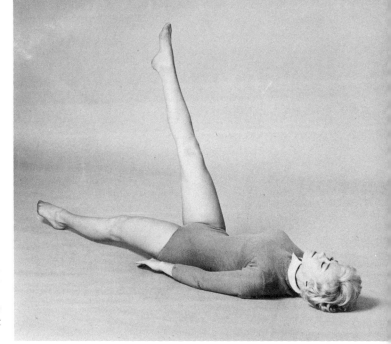

Up-and-Over

Starting position: STAND tall with the feet together. 1) Raise the arms over the head. 2) Bend forward from the waist and 3) Touch the floor with the fingers. Up and back, forward and over. The backward movement is as important as the forward bend. Get the most out of this exercise by stretching until you feel the pull on the abdominal muscles as you reach back and forward. Start with a few, ten is enough for the first time, but increase the number daily until you reach thirty.

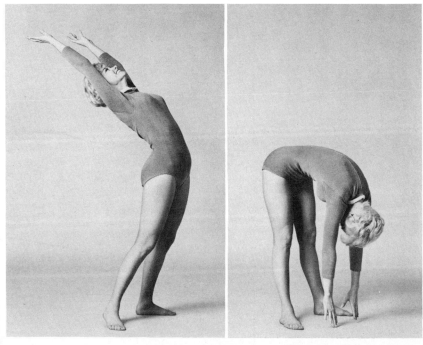

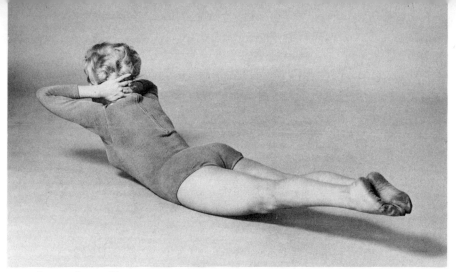

Rock and Roll

Starting position: LIE DOWN on your tummy. Clasp the hands behind the neck. 1) Lift both feet and the head slightly off the floor and 2) Rock and roll back and forth on the tummy. (This one, of course, should not be done during pregnancy.) It is hard work but this is a very effective tummy reducer.

Double Leg-Raise

Starting position: LIE DOWN on your back. You may put your hands under the hips for support or leave them on the floor alongside the body. 1) Raise the feet to a 60° angle from the floor. 2) Slowly, lower them a few inches and *hold* them there. 3) Lower feet to the floor. Repeat. This one will make you say "ouch" the first few times but it's worth it as it means the stomach is feeling the pull.

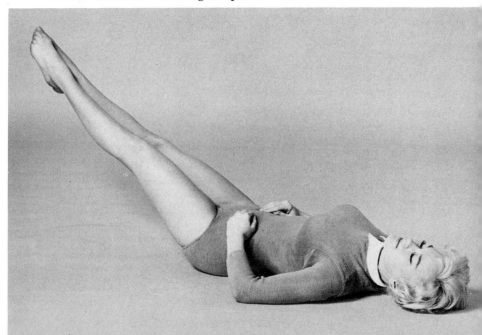

Seated Knee-Raise

Starting position: SIT in a straight chair with both feet on the floor. 1) Bring the right knee up into the tummy. 2) Hold briefly and 3) Return to floor. Repeat with the left knee. This is an easy one to do while you are telephoning or watching television. It works on the thighs as well as the tummy.

Double Knee-Raise

This is done the same way as the Seated Knee-Raise except that you raise *both* knees into the tummy at the same time. You will find it a little more difficult to get the knees all the way to the tummy, but keep trying.

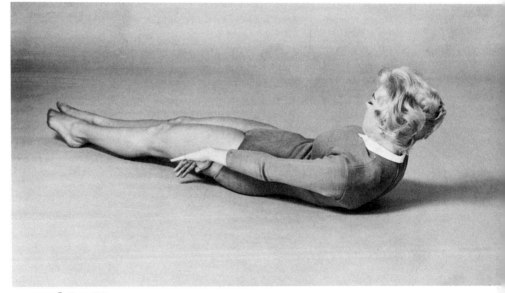

Partial Sit-Ups

Starting position: LIE DOWN on your back, with hands at sides. 1) Slowly bring the upper half of the body a few inches off the floor. 2) Slowly lower again to prone position. The slow motion gives the pull to the abdominal muscles. It is important not to overdo this one in the beginning for it creates a very strong pull. Do only one or two the first day. Add another each day as you become adjusted to the action.

Sit-and-Stand

This is a wonderful exercise for the entire lower half of the body. It flattens the tummy, reduces the hips, tightens the thighs and slims the calves.

Starting position: SIT in a straight chair with hands at the sides. 1) Rise to a standing position without using your hands for support. 2) Sit down again, without using the hands. The secret of this exercise is to do it very slowly. You mustn't jump up or plop down. The slower the movement, the greater the muscle pull.

Get in the habit of doing this whenever you sit and rise from a chair, at home or in the office.

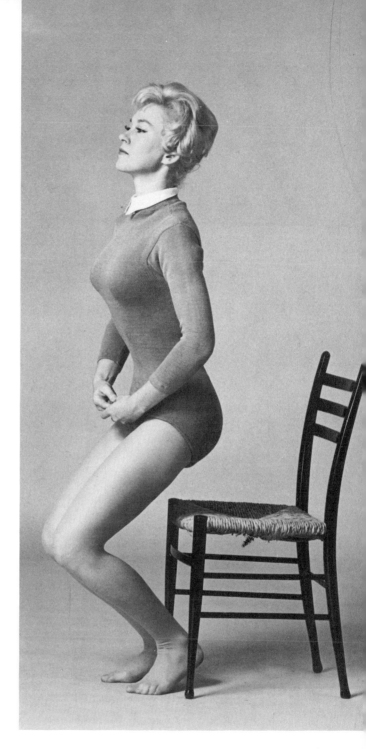

14

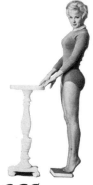

For Shapelier Legs

Exercises for the calves and ankles

Shapely legs add immeasurably to a woman's beauty. Good looking legs are not restricted to the very young. Some of the most famous legs in the world are possessed by those well over 21. The legendary Mistinguette of French music hall fame showed off her exquisite dancing legs when she had passed 70. Marlene Dietrich, the world's most glamorous grandmother, has kept her legs as perfect as ever. Betty Grable is another example of the enduring beauty of lovely legs.

Many women think that they cannot change the shape of their legs. They believe that a thick ankle or full calf must forever be their misfortune. Others think that though they may gain weight in other areas, their spindly legs are beyond correction. To these women, I want to shout an emphatic "No." You can reshape the contours of your legs just as you can re-design the rest of your body. It takes longer to get results with the calves and ankles than other areas—but it can be done if you are persistent enough.

Leg exercises must be repeated daily, without fail, to bring results. Don't look for overnight transformations—but if you seriously want to change the shape of your legs, you must start on a long-term program NOW. Eventually, improvement will appear.

One of the best exercises for the legs, from the thighs down to the ankles, is bicycling. The rotating motion brings all the leg muscles into play. Another sports activity which is excellent for the legs is swimming. I don't mean a casual dip in the surf. I mean all-out swimming with strong leg kicks. If you have access to a pool, devote a portion of your water time to holding onto the side of the pool and scissor kicking through the water.

All the calf exercises described will benefit the ankles, too. Especially valuable is the toe and heel rolling walk.

I have divided this group of exercises into Reducing and Building Up. I suggest you try all the exercises that apply to your needs and do them as often as you can.

Calf Exercises

Reducing

Starting position: STAND with your hands resting on a table or chair back. Place both feet on a book. 1) Drop the heels down to the floor. 2) Raise the body weight up onto the toes. Go up and down twenty times without stopping.

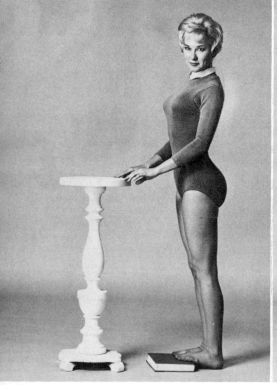 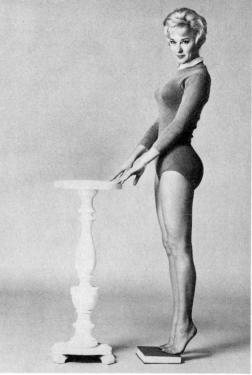

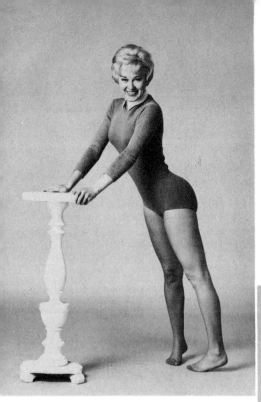

This is a three-way exercise which is very simple to do and one which brings excellent results in slimming and tightening the leg and ankles.

Starting position: STAND next to a table, with one hand resting on the table. 1) Point the toes of both feet outwards and rise up on the toes and lower ten times. 2) Turn the toes inwards and rise and lower ten times. 3) Point the toes straight ahead; rise and lower ten times. Repeat the cycle, doing ten counts in each position. Do this one as often as you possibly can.

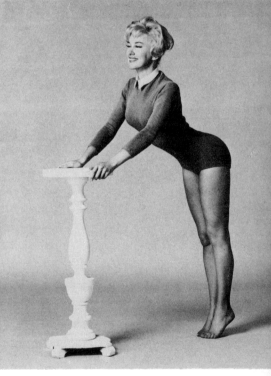

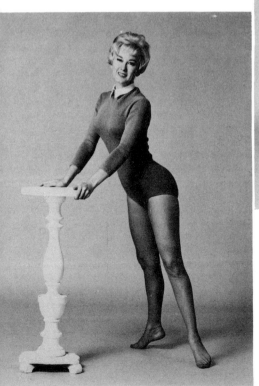

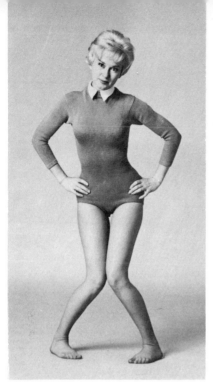

This is a leg exercise which I do frequently on television. I have had many letters telling me of the good results it brings.

Starting position: STAND with legs apart, hands on hips. 1) Squat down and turn the toes inward. 2) Walk around the room, keeping the toes in. It may look peculiar but it really works on the calves.

Shaping

TO ADD more shape to the calves, hips and thighs, try the Duck Walk. Starting position: STAND with hands on hips. 1) Bend the knees and lower the body, keeping the knees together. 2) Now, go for a walk, moving the feet straight ahead as you go.

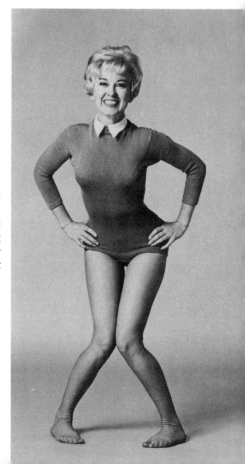

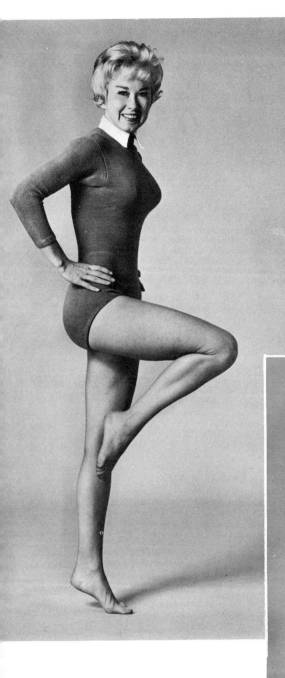

This is good for reducing and building up.

Starting position: STAND with hands on hips. 1) Step forward with the right leg, putting your weight on the toes. 2) Roll the weight from the toes to the heel. 3) Step forward with the left leg and roll the weight from the toes to the heel. This should be done as a walk, not from a stationary position. (If you bring your knees up in drum majorette style as you walk, you will help to firm the thighs, too.)

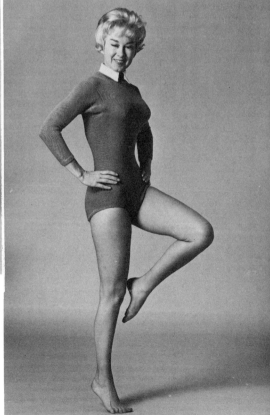

Ankle Exercises

This is easy and fun to do. I call it "Foot-Doodling." Get in the habit of practicing it whenever you are sitting down. 1) Cross the knees and with the top foot, 2) Write the alphabet in the air. Each letter gives a different pull to the ankles. You can teach your children their ABC's while you are improving your ankles.

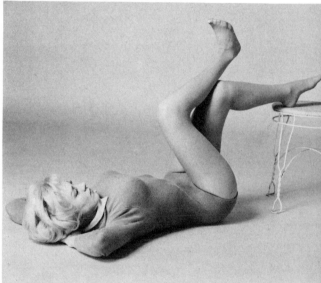

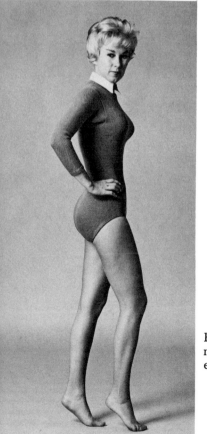

Starting position: LIE DOWN on your back with your feet resting on a chair or sofa. With the feet up and the knees crossed, 1) Draw circles in the air, using one foot, then re-crossing and using the other foot.

You may also do this without the knees crossed and using both feet at one time.

Rise up on the toes, stretching the ankle muscles. Walk on the toes for 3 to 5 minutes each morning and evening.

15

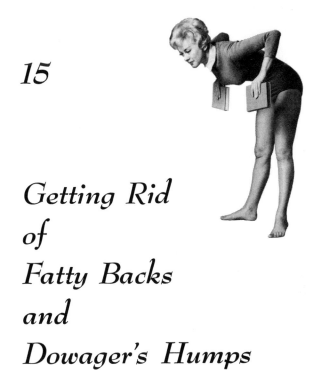

Getting Rid
of
Fatty Backs
and
Dowager's Humps

Excess fat across the back and the little bulge at the junction of the neck and shoulders which is commonly called the Dowager's Hump are beauty enemies that usually work in partnership. These are figure problems that come with the years, though a plump back can be found in overweight girls of any age. Many women would rather die than tell their ages but they shout out the march of time via these telltale figure defects.

If you have a Dowager's Hump, avoid sleeping on a pillow because this accentuates the problem. Check up on your posture habits, too. If you let your head droop forward, you may be well on your way to getting this unsightly bulge at the back of your neck. Even thin women can acquire a Dowager's Hump if they let their shoulders slump.

The following exercises will melt away the neck bulges and reduce a fatty back.

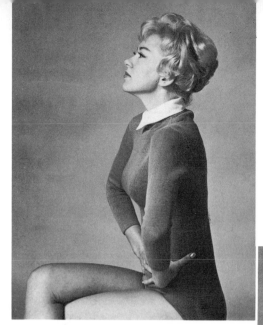

Shoulder Circles

Starting position: STAND, holding the head high. (This is something you should always do, anyway.) 1) Move the shoulders forward, 2) Up, 3) Back and 4) Down. Make these shoulder circles as big as you can, pulling hard at each turn.

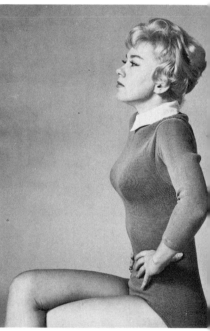

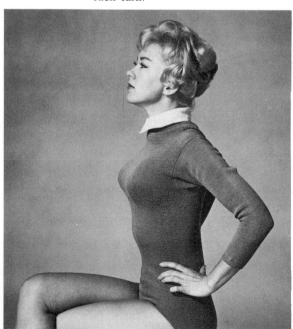

Back-Cross

Starting position: STAND tall with the hands down at the sides. 1) Raise the hands over the head and 2) Cross the hands behind the head. 3) Swing the arms down and 4) Cross the hands behind the hips. (This is the same exercise described in the Bustline chapter. It firms and lifts the bust as it works away the excess fat on the back and neck.)

Hand-Swings

Starting position: STAND tall and stretch the hands out straight in front of the body, level with the chest. 1) Swing the arms down at the sides and 2) Swing the arms as far to the back as you can. This exercise is very good for the entire upper torso.

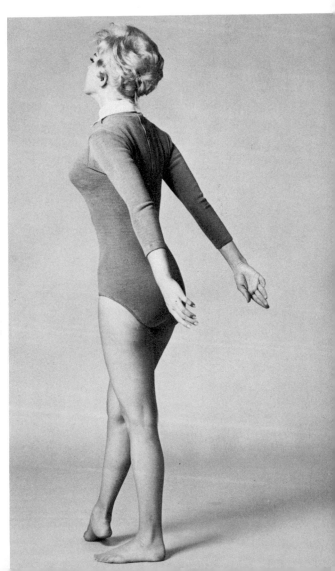

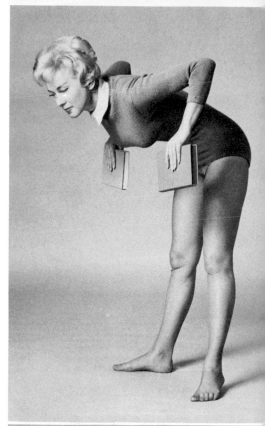

Row-the-Boat

Starting position: STAND with feet apart and bend over at the waist. Drop the arms downward towards the floor. HOLD A BOOK in each hand as the weight will increase the pull. 1) Bend the elbows and raise the books to the chest. 2) Push the books down again, straightening the arms. Pull as though you were rowing a heavy boat—the greater the pull, the better the results. Do only ten the first time, increasing daily.

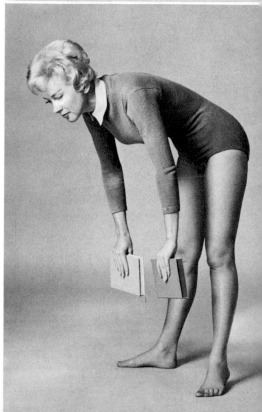

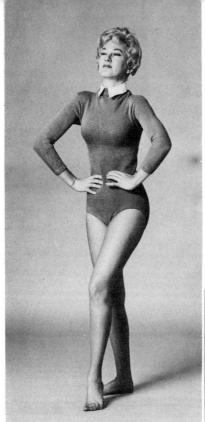

Elbow-Swings

Starting position: STAND with the hands at the waist, elbows to the sides. 1) Move the elbows forward as far as they will go. 2) Move the elbows backward as far as they will go. (This exercise is also good for the bust and upper arms.)

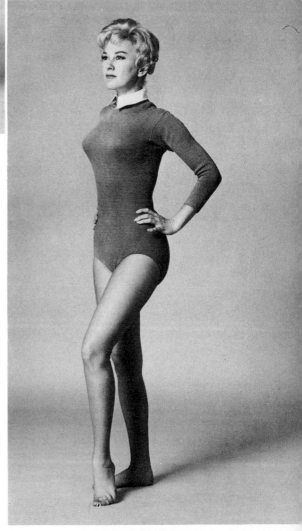

16

For Lovelier Arms

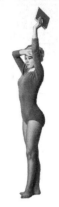

Exercises to shape, reduce, and firm the arms

Sleeveless fashions have become favorites around the clock and around the calendar. No woman can wear these styles attractively unless her arms are firm and well-shaped. A heavy arm is unsightly; a scrawny arm is unappealing and a flabby arm tells the world you are not getting any younger.

Shapeliness and firmness are the by-products of good muscle tone. The same exercises that reduce a heavy arm (when accompanied by diet) will firm a flabby arm and round out a thin arm. Few figure problems are confined to one area alone. One of the extra blessings of a regular, daily exercise program is that when you improve one part of the figure, you invariably improve other areas as well. The bustline, waist and back exercises which I have given you will also help improve the shape and tone of the arms. The arm exercises in this chapter will, in turn, improve the entire upper torso as well as the arms. As you reach up and out with the arms, you are stretching the muscles through the waist and back—and often the thighs, too. Put as much *pull* as possible into each exercise you do and you will get the maximum benefits for the entire figure.

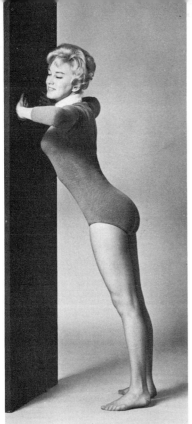

Wall Push-Outs

Starting position: STAND at arm's distance from a wall. Place the palms flat against the wall with the fingers pointing inward. 1) Push hard against the wall, bending the elbows and leaning in to the wall as you go. 2) Push away from the wall, letting the arms carry the body weight back to an upright position.

This is excellent for reducing heavy arms and for firming flabby ones.

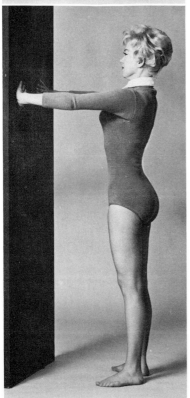

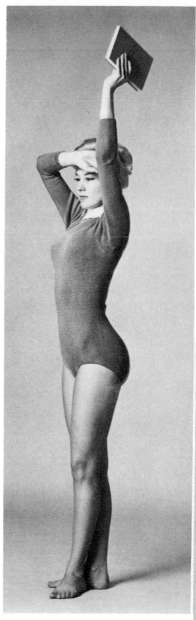

The Book-Reach

Starting position: STAND tall with a book in one hand. Raise the arm straight up over the head. Grasp the raised arm with the other hand. 1) Bend the raised arm at the elbow and 2) Straighten the arm above the head. Fling the book up and down with strong movements. Repeat for ten times with each arm. Feel the stretch through your ribcage as the book goes up and down.

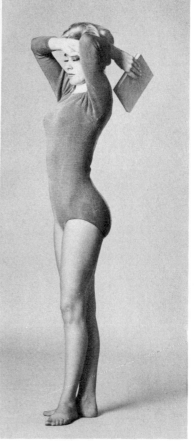

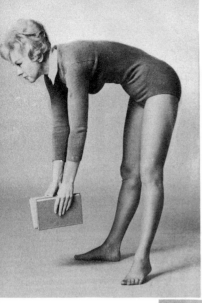

The Back-Reach

Starting position: STAND, holding a book in each hand. Bend over at the waist and let the arms drop down towards the floor. 1) Fling the books out toward the back and 2) return to the front of the body. Really push out hard as you fling them back and forth. This is good for the bustline as well as the arms.

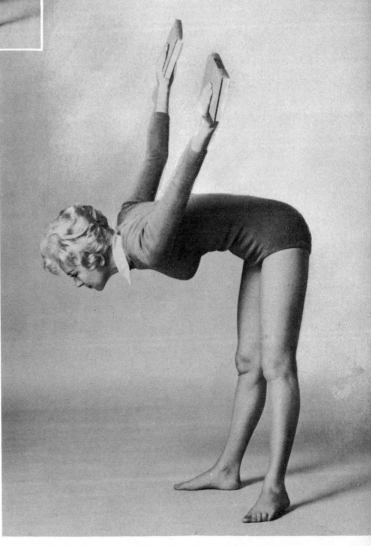

Arm Pushups

Starting position: SIT on the floor with the arms stiff and the palms facing the front of the body. With the hips remaining firmly on the floor, 1) Lower the upper half of the body, bending the elbows as you go down. 2) Raise up, straightening the arms. Start with ten of these and increase gradually.

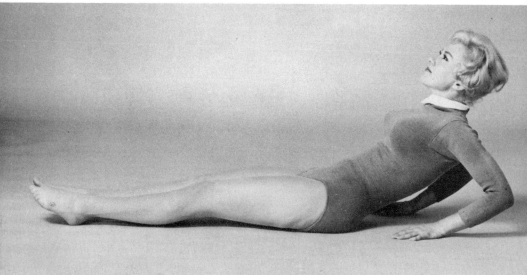

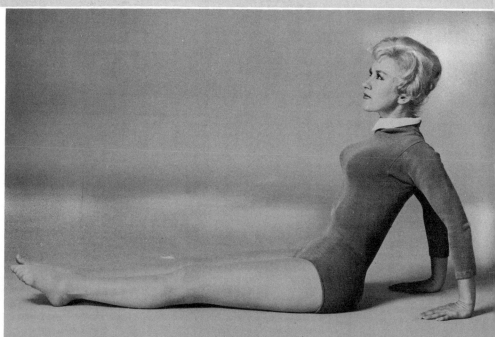

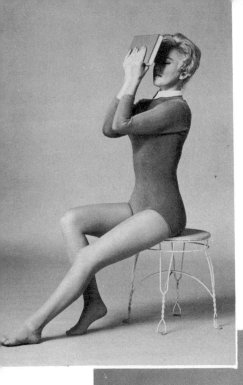

Front-Reach

Starting position: SEATED or STANDING. Hold a book with both hands against the forehead. 1) Extend the book straight out and 2) return to forehead. Remember that the more you put into each exercise, the more you will get out of it. Really push in and out as you move the book to get the best results.

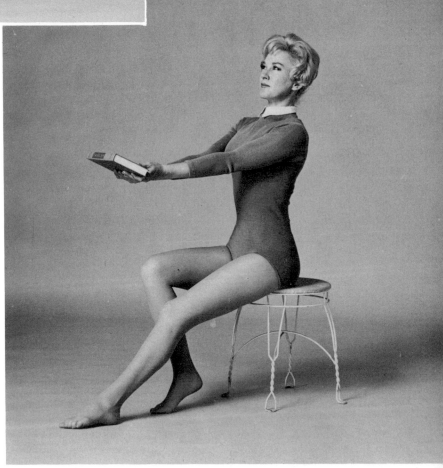

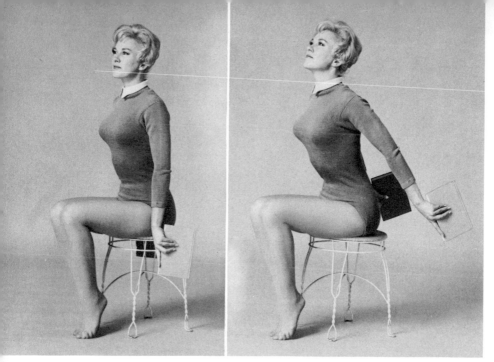

Seated Back-Reach

Here is an exercise you can do almost anytime you think of it, in the office or around the house. Use a book in each hand if you have some handy. If not, do it with the hands free. 1) Drop the arms at the sides of the chair and 2) swing them backwards, keeping the elbows stiff. 3) Return and swing again. This is very good for the bustline, too.

The Criss-Cross

I am repeating this exercise because it is very good for the arms as well as for the bustline and the back.

Starting position: STAND straight with the arms at the sides. 1) Raise the arms above the head and cross the hands behind the head. 2) Lower the arms to the sides and cross the hands behind the hips. Start with ten and gradually add a few more each day.

Arm Circles

This is another repeat. It is excellent for the bust and the back, as well as the arms.

Starting position: STAND with the arms out at the sides level with the shoulders. 1) Draw rapid circles with both hands at the same time. You should feel the pull starting from the wrists and going right up through the arms, the chest and the back. Start with ten and increase daily.

17

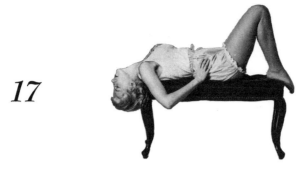

A Youthful Neckline

Goodbye to double chins and crêpe necks

Nothing tells your age like a double chin or loose, crêpy throat. Jewelry and scarves may cover up an aging neckline but there are many times when you must go without the camouflage. A double chin, on the other hand, is impossible to conceal.

Why not cure these beauty faults with exercise? The following group is easy to do and will prevent as well as cure the problems.

A special word about double chins. Many women think they are hereditary and that nothing can be done about them. On the contrary, most double chins come from overweight and faulty posture. Diet and exercise will take care of the first cause. Holding your head high and keeping your chin parallel to the floor will go a long way toward correcting the second.

To keep your neckline more youthful, massage it with an upward stroke frequently. Whenever you use cleansing cream, work it in from the base of the neck and firmly push the neck with an upward motion. This will help to keep the tissues firm. Downward strokes loosen the tissue and make it saggy.

The Chin Lift

This, as you will remember, is one of my Basic Six exercises which I believe every woman should do every day. It is easier to prevent a problem than to cure it—although this exercise will do both. 1) Throw the head back and open the mouth. 2) Bring the lower lip on top of the upper lip. Push the chin up toward the ceiling.

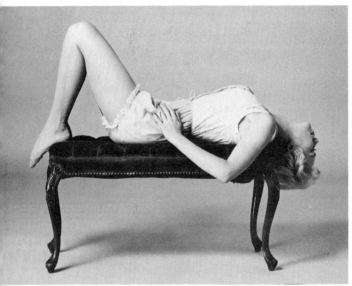

Head-Lift

Starting position: LIE down on your sofa or bed. Drop the head down over the edge. Lying on your back, 1) Bring the head up until the chin touches the chest.

You wouldn't think that an exercise that gets rid of a double chin could also help reduce the tummy, but this one does. As you practice it, you will feel the pull on the stomach muscles as the head is raised.

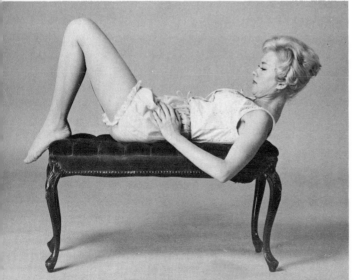

Head Circles

Starting position: SIT OR STAND and tilt the head back. 1) Circle the head from top to side, back to side, bringing it as far in each direction as you can.

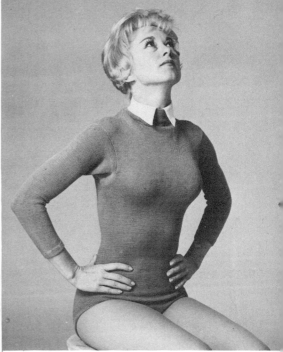

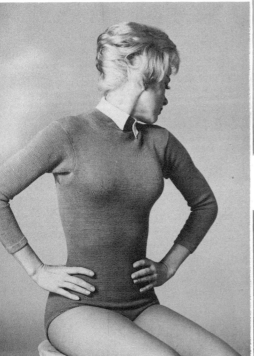

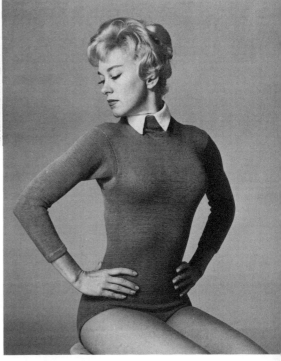

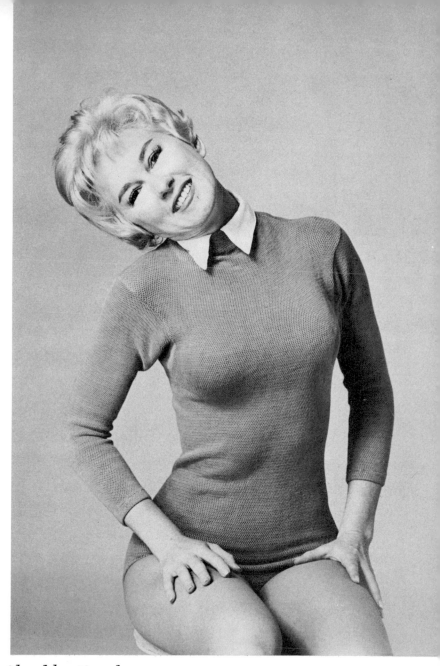

Shoulder-Touch
Starting position: SIT OR STAND. *Without turning the head* 1) Drop
the head to the left and try to touch the left shoulder. 2) Drop the head
to the right and try to touch the right shoulder. Let the head and the neck
do the work. Don't raise the shoulders to meet the head. It is the pull on
the neck muscles we are after.

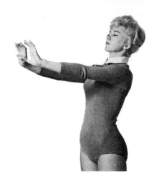

18

For Graceful Hands
and Slender Wrists

Your hands and wrists are as much a part of your figure as
your other proportions. We are striving for over-all perfection
and the hands play an important part in creating that impression of graceful, feminine beauty.

Extra weight settles in the hands just as it does elsewhere.
Have you noticed how many women's wedding rings have
become buried in a well of flesh on their fingers? The slender,
tapering fingers on which these rings were once placed have
grown fat with the years, just as other parts of the figure have
swelled with time.

Graceful, well-shaped hands enhance your femininity. Hand-
grooming (manicures, lotioning, etc.) is not enough to make
your hands beautiful. The shape and the quality of gesture is
equally important.

Take a look at your own hands and wrists. Are they well-
shaped and gracefully expressive? Hand exercises will make
them that way . . . and they are the easiest of all exercises
to do, for they can be fitted into almost any portion of your
daily schedule. Hand exercises can be done while waiting in a
car, talking on the telephone, watching television or during
other odd moments during the day when the hands are free.
Try doing some of them to music. It's easy and fun, too.

An extra tip on hand beauty: When you apply hand lotion
(which you should do regularly several times a day to keep

187

the hands smooth and soft) work the cream in with firm, massaging strokes. Pull out the fingers one by one as you apply the lotion. Work it into the wrists well—pulling the skin downward from the hands.

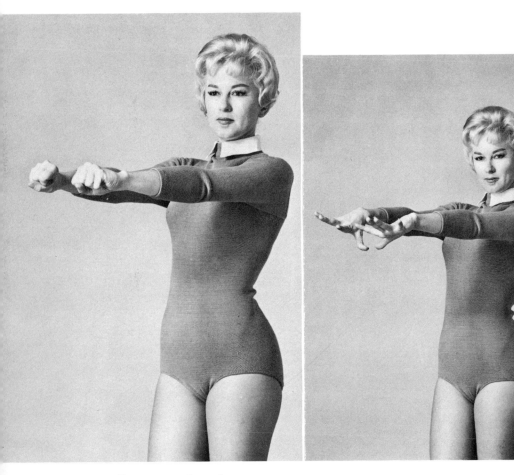

The Fist Clench

Flexibility is the key to graceful hands. The more you stretch the fingers, the more supple they become. The fist clench involves two motions. 1) Make tight fists with your hands and 2) Open the fists and stretch the fingers out to full length.

The Wrist Shake

1) Pull the hands into the chest and 2) shake vigorously. The action should all come from the wrists when you shake.

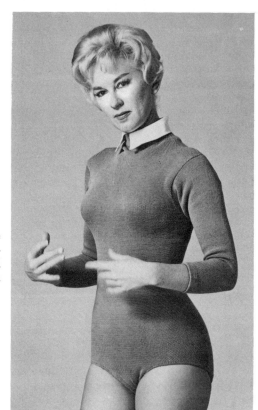

The Swan

Think of the graceful, sliding motion of swans as you do this exercise. Starting position: Elbows bent and palms skyward at shoulder level. 1) Leading with the wrists, bring the palms forward and 2) leading with the wrists, return the palms to the shoulders. Let the wrists flip over as they reach the forward position; flip back again when they reach the shoulders. Remember the curve of the swan's neck as the wrists shift position.

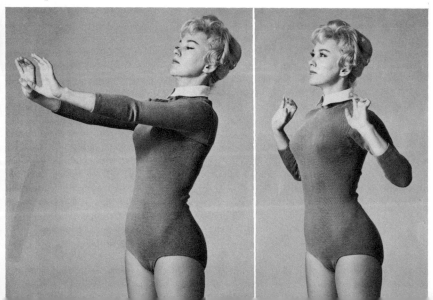

Side-Swans

Starting position: Extend the arms full length from the sides at shoulder level. 1) Leading with the wrists, push the hands out to the sides and 2) Leading with the wrists, return the hands to the shoulders. This one improves the shape of the arms as well as the wrists and hands.

Hawaii

These are the Swans again but in Hawaiian disguise. 1) Leading with the wrists, cross the palms in front of the chest. 2) Flip the wrists and return. (I always hum "Sweet Leilani" to myself when I do this exercise.) The graceful movement of the hands to and fro is characteristic of the Hawaiian dances in which the hands play a vital role in telling the story of the music.

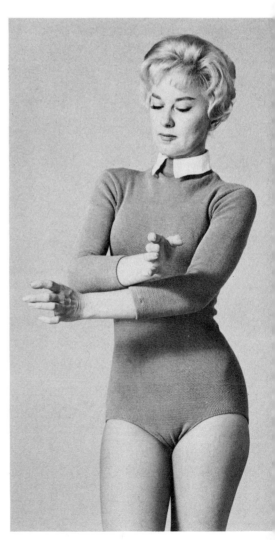

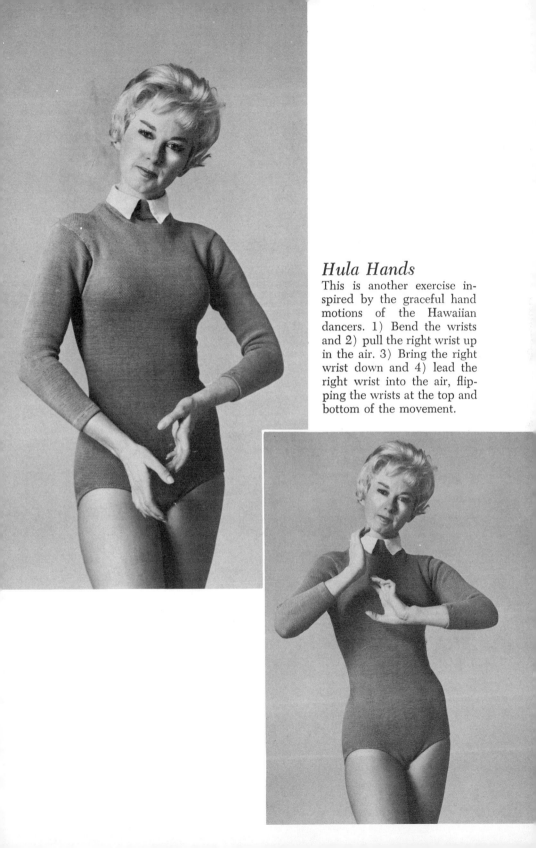

Hula Hands

This is another exercise inspired by the graceful hand motions of the Hawaiian dancers. 1) Bend the wrists and 2) pull the right wrist up in the air. 3) Bring the right wrist down and 4) lead the right wrist into the air, flipping the wrists at the top and bottom of the movement.

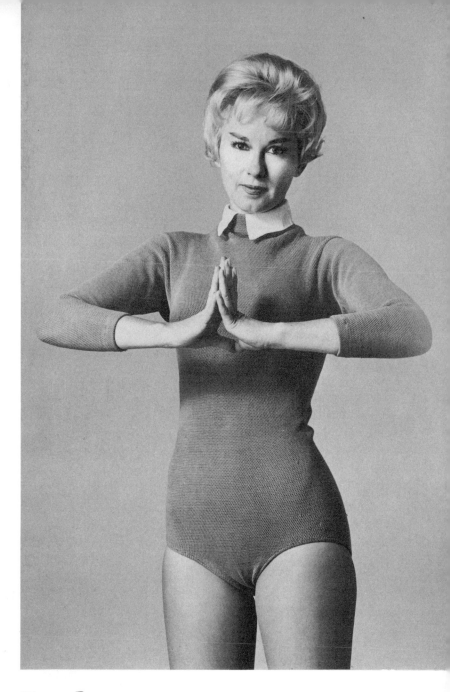

Finger-Bounce

This exercise will greatly increase the flexibility of the hands. 1) Place the fingers of the hands together and 2) bounce the palms together in a rhythmic movement.

19

Facial Exercises

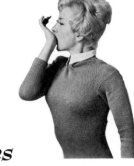

Keeping the face firm and youthful

The facial muscles need tightening and toning just as the rest of body muscles do. Many women complain that their faces get haggard looking when they lose weight. Others say the first pound they gain seems to settle in their faces—giving them a plump look. Whichever seems to be your problem, these facial exercises will correct it if you do a few of them daily. They will keep the face firm and youthful looking; guard against aging lines, wrinkles and skin folds—and improve the skin tone and the complexion.

To increase the circulation around the mouth and give your lips a fresh natural color, try this beauty tip: Press a very warm towel or washcloth against the lips and leave it on until it gets cool. This is a good procedure to follow before applying make-up.

Chin and Jaw Firmer

Take a roll of gauze about one inch in thickness. 1) Place the gauze roll in one side of the mouth and chew. 2) Shift the gauze to the other side of the mouth and chew. Don't force it; move the jaw up and down in easy chewing motions. Chew on one side for ten times—alternate to the other for ten times. This will firm the tissue of the jaw and lower cheek, correcting the sag that comes with weight loss.

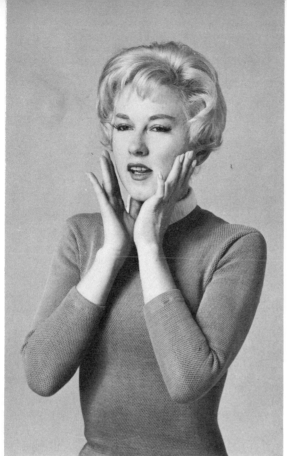

Jaw Twist

Starting position: Place the hands on either side of the face, just lightly touching the jaw. 1) Twist the jaw (not the head nor the hands) to the left until it touches the left hand. 2) Twist the jaw to the right until it touches the right hand.

Cheek Reducer

If your cheeks are too full, practice this exercise regularly to reduce them. 1) With the mouth closed and the teeth slightly apart, *suck* the cheeks between the teeth. Relax, repeat. You will literally suck away the extra fatty tissue that puffs out a fat cheek.

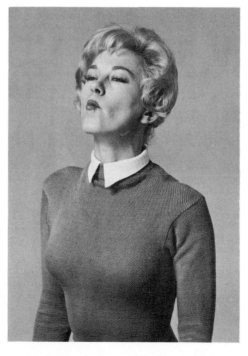

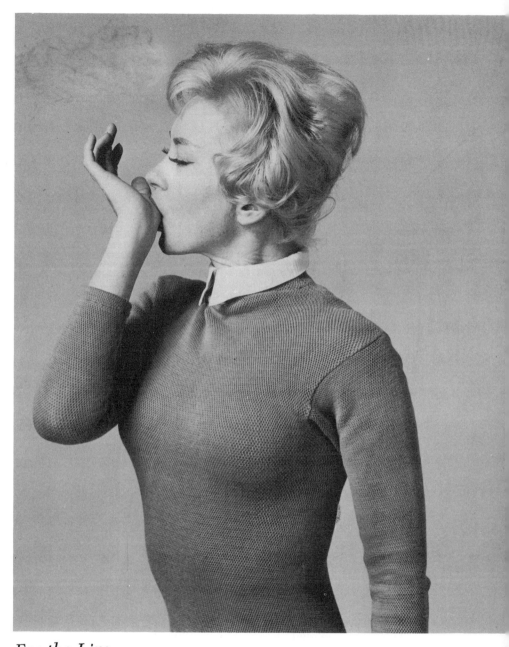

For the Lips

If you want more appealing lips, try this one. It will develop a thin mouth into fuller contours and keep full lips at their loveliest.

1) With the lips slightly parted, suck against the heel of the hand.

20

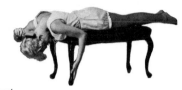

You Can Even
Exercise
Your Hair!

How to stimulate growth
and improve the texture

Massaging and brushing are forms of exercising the hair. Massage stimulates the scalp and improves the circulation which, in turn, encourages the growth of the hair. Regular brushing helps the flow of the natural oils through the hair, improving the lustre and texture.

When massaging the scalp or brushing the hair, it is always preferable to work from a prone position. Lie down on a couch or bed and let the head hang over the edge. This sends the blood to the roots of the hair and aids the circulation.

All three of these hair exercises will improve the complexion and skin tone as well as the hair. I also find them excellent for relieving tension and fatigue.

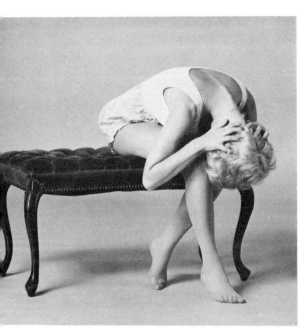

Massaging

To massage the scalp, start from the nape of the neck and work with firm circular finger motions from the neck to the forehead. It is the scalp that should move in each position, not the fingers.

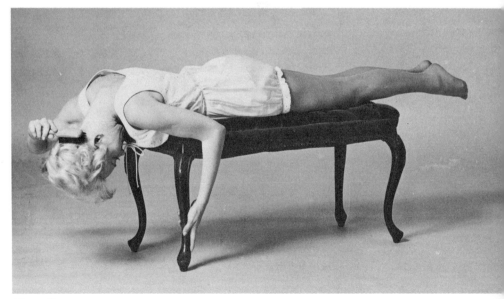

Brushing

Use a firm brush with natural bristles. Lie across the bed with the head over the edge, face down. Brush from the nape of the neck forward.

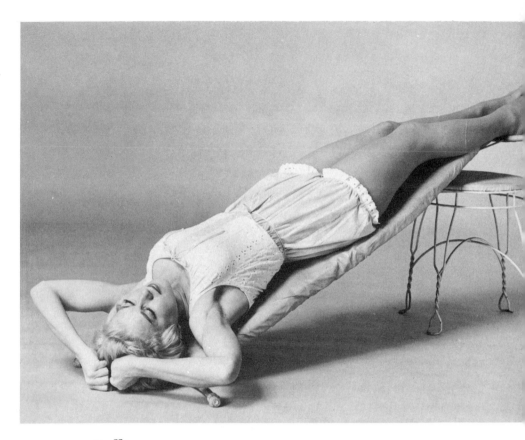

Pulling

To stimulate growth, lie on a slanting board, head down and feet up. (I use an ironing board for this.) Grasp a generous section of the hair with each hand and pull. Work systematically up and down over the scalp so that each section of the hair is exercised.

21

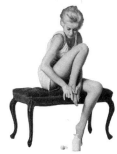

Let's Play Footsie!

Exercises for the feet
and arches

No other part of the body suffers the wear and tear the feet do. We crowd them into tight, pointed shoes; give them the burden of our body weight to carry day in and day out—yet seldom think to pamper them with special exercises and care to restore their strength.

To keep your best foot forward, follow these foot care rules:

1. Remove your shoes as often as possible and stretch out your toes, flex your arches and rotate your ankles.

2. Be sure your stocking size is ample. A short stocking will crowd the toes and impair the circulation.

3. Change your heel heights often. Regular changing from high to lower heels pulls and strengthens the calf and ankle muscles.

4. If you wear pointed toes (and who doesn't these days?), make sure you are fitted with a shoe size that is long enough to avoid crowding the toes.

5. Treat yourself to a good foot-soak as often as possible. Soak the feet first in warm water (the hotter, the better)

—then in cold water. This will improve the circulation and firm the foot tissues. It also provides soothing relief to aching feet.

6. Rub the feet with body lotion after bathing. Pull the toes one at a time. Rub the soles and arches with a firm, circular motion.

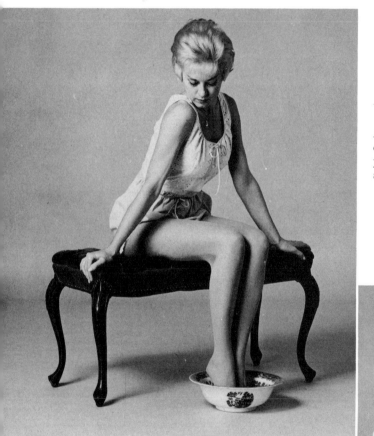

Alternating hot and cold foot soaks will improve the circulation and firm the tissues.

Massage the feet with body lotion after bathing. Use firm, circular motions.

22

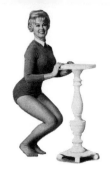

Exercises to Do During Pregnancy and After the Baby Comes

So many women write to me asking what exercises they can do while they are pregnant and how they can get their figures back after the baby is born. Unless there is a special problem, doctors agree that exercising regularly throughout pregnancy keeps the mother-to-be in better health, shape and spirits. The more limber and supple the muscles are kept, the easier the delivery. And—the easier it will be for the new mother to regain her figure afterwards.

It is very important that you consult your own doctor before starting an exercise program during pregnancy. He may have special cautions to suggest. Show him this book and get his approval for the exercises you intend to follow.

The average mother-to-be can follow any of the exercises I have outlined WITH THESE EXCEPTIONS: However, your own doctor is the one to give the go ahead signal to your exercise routine.

1. NO overhead reaches
2. NO bends more than 45% from the waist
3. NO leg bounces
4. NO more than slight waist circles

The "Squats" which I have described in Chapter 11 are especially good for most women during pregnancy. They limber and strengthen the pelvic muscles and keep the lower torso limber. Let me remind you how they are done:

The Squats

Starting position: STAND with one hand resting on the back of a chair or table; the other hand at the waist. 1) Slowly, lower the body from a standing position to a sitting (or "squatting") position. 2) Slowly, rise to a standing position again. Ten of these every day during pregnancy is recommended—but check with your doctor first.

The First Three Days
After Childbirth

These exercises can be done on the hospital bed, before you are allowed to stand or walk. Show them to your doctor and get his approval in case there are special reasons for restricting your activity during this period.

First Day

Lie flat on your bed and push the toes into the end of the bed. Do five in the morning and five in the afternoon. Increase to ten on the second and third days.

Second Day

Lying on your back with the legs extended and the knees straight, 1) Raise one leg to the count of 1-2-3 and 2) Lower the leg to the count of 4-5-6. Alternate and raise the other leg to the same count. Do five with each leg the first day, work gradually up to ten. Continue this for several weeks after the baby is born.

Third Day

Bed Sit-Ups. Lying on your back, raise yourself to a sitting position. Extend your arms and touch your toes. Do five in the morning and five in the afternoon. Increase to ten and add more as you feel stronger. This exercise will help the abdominal muscles regain their elasticity—tightening and flattening the tummy.

Home from the Hospital

Once home from the hospital, you are ready to resume a moderate daily exercise routine. Continue the bed exercises and when you are feeling stronger, add two exercises each for the bust, the tummy, the hips and thighs—and any other special area which requires improving. Start with five counts for each exercise and add a few each day.

In addition, do the Camel Walk to strengthen the abdominal wall and help speed the return of the uterus to its normal position.

The Camel Walk

Starting position: Get down on the floor and raise up on your hands and feet, keeping the hips as high in the air as possible. 1) Walk around the room in this position until you feel any signs of straining. Increase the walking time daily.

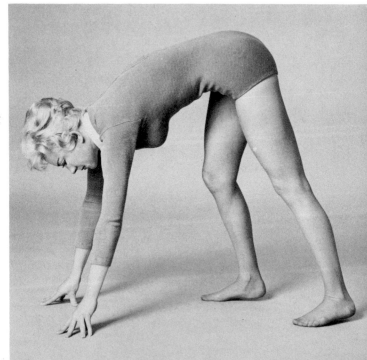

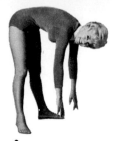

23

Relieving Tension

Do you often find yourself grumpy and on edge—easily upset by the most trivial misfortunes? You are suffering from tension —one of the most common ailments of our times. As the pressures of our daily lives increase, we find that tension mounts and we have a difficult time relaxing. With nervous tension comes a constriction of the body muscles. This makes us feel tied up in knots—which, in a sense, we are—for the muscles are over-tensed. Exercise will loosen them up and relieve the pressure on the nerve ends. The body relaxes and resumes its normal calm.

Whenever I have trouble getting to sleep at night, I do a few exercises. They relieve the tension and prepare me for a good, restful sleep.

The next time you feel tense and upset, take time out to try these relaxers.

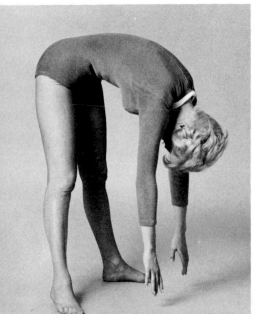

The Bounce

Starting position: STAND and bend over from the hips. Keep the knees straight but let the rest of the body dangle like a rag doll. 1) Bounce up and down from the hips; let the body go up and down like a ball on a rubber string. You can bounce away the blues— bounce away backaches— even bounce away a burst of temper.

Deep Breathing

Often, tension is the result of lack of sufficient oxygen in the lungs. Deep breathing will lessen fatigue and give a refreshing lift to the spirits as well as the system.

Starting position: STAND tall with your hands on your hips. 1) Take a deep breath and 2) Rise up on your toes. 3) Hold your breath and stay on your toes for about 20 seconds. 4) Slowly exhale as you come back down again. If you can do this one in front of an open window or out of doors, so much the better.

Head-and-Knee Touch

Starting position: SIT on the floor with your legs apart. With your hands at the waist, 1) Bend the head forward and touch the right knee with it. 2) Bring the head back then repeat, touching the left knee. (It will help your spirits to know that you are slimming your waistline while you are relieving your tensions.)

Shoulder Shakes

Do this while sitting or standing. 1) Bend the shoulders forward and 2) Bend the shoulders back. Repeat at least ten times. This is a good exercise for anyone who sits at a desk all day long. It relieves the tension in the shoulders. It is also excellent to do at frequent intervals on a long driving trip.

Arm Stretches

This exercise is good to use when you go to bed. It pulls out the kinks and gets you ready for peaceful dreams. LIE on your back with your arms at your sides. 1) Raise the arms and extend them straight over your head. 2) Climb with the arms, giving them a good stretch.

All-over Relaxers

One of the best ways to relax the body is first to achieve maximum tension, then quickly release the tension completely. Instead of counting sheep, try this before going to sleep: LIE DOWN in bed and 1) Pull in all the muscles of the arms and upper torso. Clench your fists; pull in your elbows; tighten the shoulders and hunch your back. 2) Hold the tension to the count of five, then let it go.

Do the same with the lower half of the body: Tighten the stomach; contract the buttocks; pull in the leg and foot muscles. Hold to a count of five, then let go.

Baths for Relaxing

A warm bath before retiring relaxes tired nerves and soothes aching muscles. If you are tense, but must get ready for guests or an evening out—take a warm bath but follow it with a cool shower. The cool rinse will wake you up and make you feel ready for fun.

24

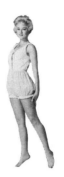

How to Get Up
in the Morning
(and Feel Better
All Day Long)

"Oh, how I hate to get up in the morning" used to be my theme song until I learned the right way to get out of bed. I used to force myself to jump up at the buzz of the alarm clock—but I never really came to life until I was halfway through my breakfast. Now I have discovered that a few exercises in bed when I awaken make all the difference in my early morning attitude.

This is the ideal time for you to start your fifteen-minutes-a-day exercise routine. Follow it with a bracing shower and nourishing breakfast—and you will look and feel your best all day long.

Have you ever watched a cat or a dog wake up? They never jump right up from a sound sleep. They stretch each muscle in their bodies very carefully before getting on their feet. We humans can learn a valuable lesson from our four-footed friends. Here are my Waker-Uppers:

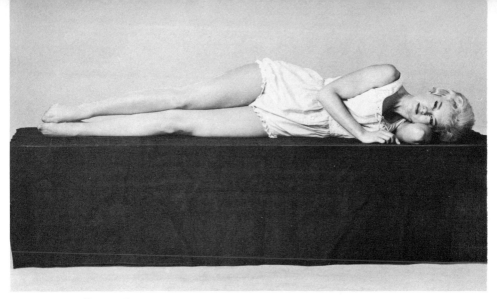

Step One

While lying down, stretch the body out to full length. Spread your toes and extend your legs; stretch the torso.

Step Two

Now, turn on your side and double your knees in to the body. Bend your back into the knees. Then stretch out again, making yourself as long and tall as you can. Repeat two or three times.

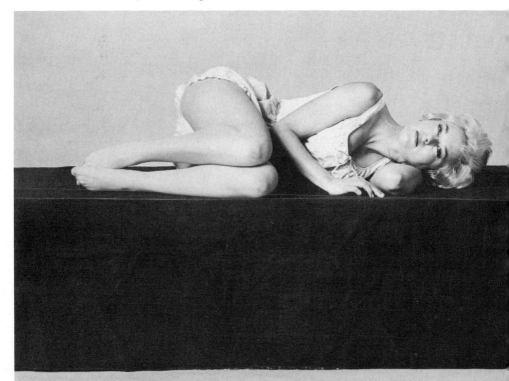

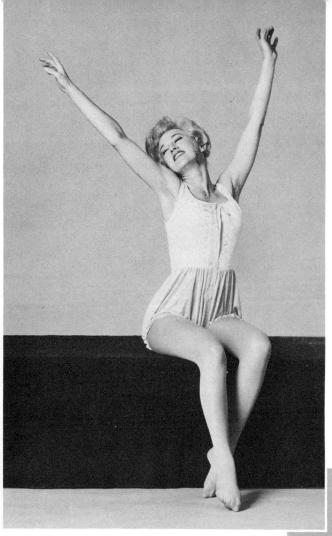

Step Three

By now, you are ready to sit up. Swing your legs over the edge of the bed, and in a sitting position, stretch your hands over your head; bend at the waist and touch your toes down there on the floor. Repeat two or three times.

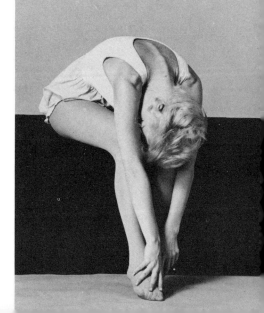

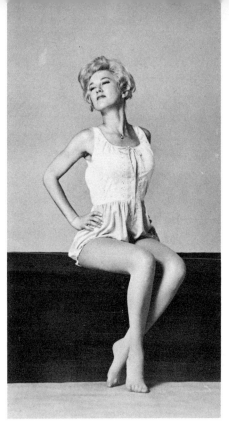

Step Four

While still sitting, put your hands at your waist and bend the elbows forward, then stretch the elbows back. Return and relax. Repeat two or three times.

Step Five

These should have been enough to put you on your feet. While still barefooted, rise and walk around the room on your tip-toes. I like to do this with my arms stretched upwards for waistline pull.

This is the ideal time for you to start your fifteen-minutes-a-day exercise routine. Follow it with a bracing shower and nourishing breakfast and you will look and feel your best all day long.

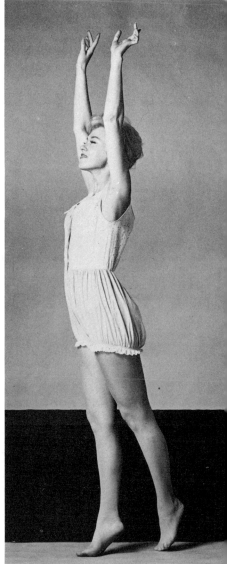

25

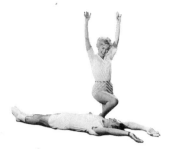

For Men Only

About one-half of all the men in their thirties are at least ten per cent above their most desirable weight, and one quarter of them are twenty per cent above. This is disturbing news not only for the American male but for the ladies, too, who like to see a man with old-fashioned muscles once in a while. All too often, by the time a man reaches his late thirties his muscles have turned to flab, his waist is ringed with the familiar spare tire, and he carries a paunch below it. A sudden dash to catch the 8:03 or a session of furniture moving leaves him panting like a coon hound in August.

Lose this extra freight, tone up those muscles and you'll be surprised at how youthful and vigorous you'll feel. Don't use a sedentary job as an excuse. What could be more sedentary, on the face of it, than the work of a judge or a legislator? Yet Supreme Court Justice William O. Douglas, in his sixties, enjoys a stamina and physique that a man thirty-five years his junior could envy. A believer in the vigorous life, Justice Douglas is famous for his long walking trips and mountain climbing. Senator Theodore Green of Rhode Island, slim and hardy in his nineties, retained sufficient vigor of mind and body to head the Senate Foreign Relations Committee and was often seen walking long distances around Washington and scampering up the Capitol steps like a fifteen-year-old. The late King Gustavus of Sweden played tennis almost daily until he was past the ninety mark. And let's not forget the young and vital Bob Cummings who is over fifty but looks half his age.

Football, baseball, hockey and other vigorous, even violent, sports are fine for high school and college boys, but they have little "carry-over value" for later life. Golf, tennis and swimming are activities that the average person can continue to enjoy, even into old age. If you've reached adulthood without learning any of these, don't despair. It's never too late to learn and as psychologists tell us continually, learning something new is the best antidote for aging.

How to Get Rid of That Paunch

No matter what sports you pursue, however, you can keep healthier and slimmer by supplementing them with fifteen minutes of daily exercise. Many men who have seen my television program have written in asking whether I have any special recommendations for masculine exercises. There are four which I think every man should do every day to keep himself trim and well-conditioned.

For just one week do the four exercises which are illustrated here. It's best to do them as soon as you get out of bed in the morning. During the first week, do ten repetitions of each exercise. Follow up with a brisk shower and a balanced breakfast. You'll start your day feeling younger, more vital and aglow than you've felt in years.

These four exercises are to men what the Basic Six exercises are to women. They are basic toners and trimmers. They improve the circulation by helping the heart to pump the blood out to all the parts of the body.

The Floor Touch and the Seated Toe Touch will get rid of the folds of fat around the waistline. They slim, and tighten the abdomen. The midriff is a man's "youthline"—any bulges in the areas above, around and below the waist add years to a man's appearance. A man can lose ten, twenty or more pounds by following a reducing diet, and yet retain his old problem paunch. These two exercises, done regularly, will trim off the waistline bulges, flatten the abdomen and pull in the paunch.

Pushups keep the arms tight and limber. No sag can settle on an upper arm that is exercised regularly. This exercise also builds up the chest and develops the muscles in the shoulders, trimming away the flab in these areas.

Knee Bends tighten, form and strengthen the leg and thigh muscles. They are extremely beneficial in counteracting the effects of too much sitting, either at a desk or in a car. They restore the muscle tone and put a youthful bounce in a man's stride.

These four exercises are all that most men need to keep them in good form throughout a lifetime. It is the regular daily repetition of these exercises which pays the dividends of a younger appearance, increased vigor and greater physical endurance.

After the first week, you will be able to add more repetitions of each exercise to your daily routine. Add a few counts each day until you reach a total of at least 30 repetitions for each exercise. How many more you do from that point is up to you. As long as you don't over-tire yourself in the beginning and work up gradually, you can do as many as you like.

Trimmers and Toners for Men

In these photos the gentleman who was kind enough to pose with me is Mr. William A. Waddick, prominent Indianapolis attorney, who keeps himself trim with regular exercise.

Ray Conolly

THE FLOOR TOUCH: (for slimming and tightening the abdomen, getting rid of the "spare tire")

Stand with the feet slightly apart. 1) Raise the hands above the head and 2) Bend from the waist and 3) Touch the floor with t h e fingers. Keep the legs straight throughout to get the maximum pull in the thigh and calf muscles.

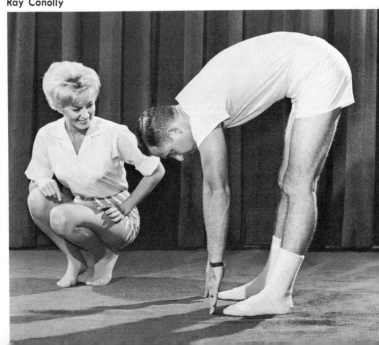

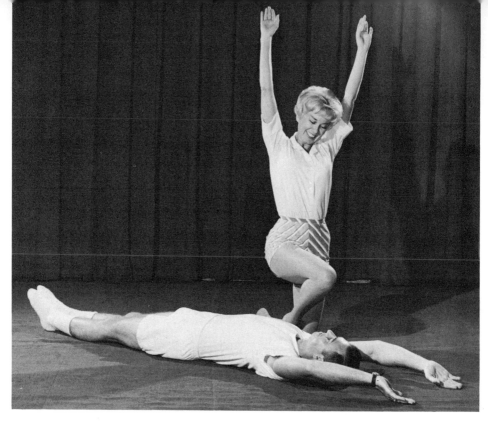

SEATED TOE TOUCH: (for trimming down the paunch, narrowing the midriff)

Stretch out full length on the floor. Point the toes. Extend the arms straight out above the head.

Raise the arms from the floor, rise to a sitting position and touch the toes.

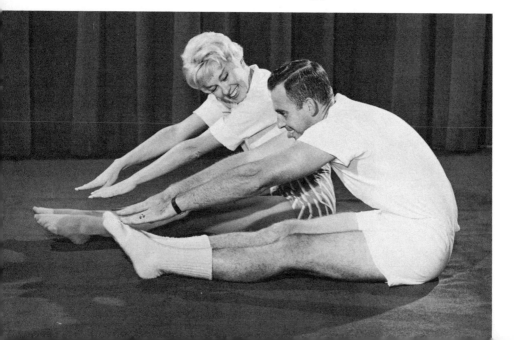

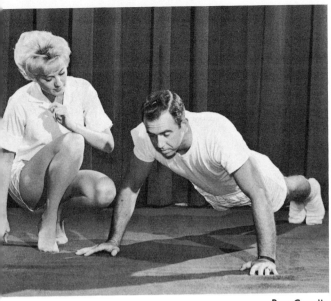

PUSHUPS: (for developing the chest and arms; getting rid of flabby fat on the arms, shoulders and upper back.)

Rest your weight between your toes and your hands, keeping your arms rigid and your body off the floor. Bend the elbows and lower the body slowly until it almost reaches the floor and then raise it again to the starting position.

Ray Conolly

DEEP KNEE BENDS: (for strengthening and trimming the thighs and calves) Stand with the feet slightly apart. Keep the back straight and slowly lower to a squatting position. Rise slowly and repeat.

Note: You can keep the arms straight out in front of you or tuck the hands into the waist while doing this. Choose whichever position gives you better balance.

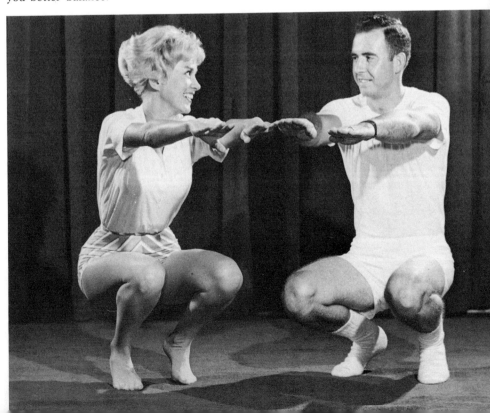

And What Do You Weigh, Sir?

If you haven't checked in at the scales recently, why not do so now and see how your weight compares with the desirable levels for your height and body frame. This chart may have a few surprises in store for you as it is based on the recent findings concerning weight and health. The old charts listed *average* weights. Surveys made by life insurance companies in the past few years show that the lowest mortality rate occurs among people who are from ten to twenty pounds *under the average* weight for their height. This chart, compiled by the Metropolitan Life Insurance Company, lists your most *desirable* weight, which is considerably below the average. You will be healthier and live longer if your weight is kept within the limits specified on this chart. (Need I add that you will also look younger and more attractive when you shed those excess pounds?)

DESIRABLE WEIGHTS FOR MEN

	FRAME SIZE		
Height (in shoes)	*Small*	*Medium*	*Large*
5′2″	112-120	118-129	126-141
5′3″	115-123	121-133	129-144
5′4″	118-126	124-136	132-148
5′5″	121-129	127-139	135-152
5′6″	124-133	130-143	138-156
5′7″	128-137	134-147	142-161
5′8″	132-141	138-152	147-166
5′9″	136-146	142-156	151-170
5′10″	140-150	146-160	157-174
5′11″	144-154	150-165	159-179
6′	148-158	154-170	164-184
6′1″	152-162	158-175	168-189
6′2″	156-167	162-180	173-194
6′3″	160-171	167-185	178-199
6′4″	164-175	172-190	182-204

Your daily exercises will keep you well toned and trim, but they won't take off weight. A cut in your daily calorie intake is necessary to get rid of the extra pounds. It is not hard to reduce, once you make up your mind to do it, and the promise of a handsome, healthy body should provide all the encouragement you need to get you started.

You can lose ten pounds easily, painlessly and permanently in only thirty days by keeping a careful count of your calories. If you have more weight than this to lose, I suggest you consult your doctor to find out if there is any medical cause involved. A thorough medical checkup every year is a good idea anyway, regardless of your weight. Tragic illnesses can often be prevented if they are detected in time.

One of the easiest ways to reduce without making any major changes in your present eating habits is to cut out some of the obvious "extras" which increase your daily calorie total but do not really add to the general pleasure of eating. For instance, if you go without rolls and butter with your lunch and dinner, you save about 150 calories at each of those meals. If you substitute a fresh fruit (approximately 50 calories) for a heavier dessert (pie, 125 calories; cake, 225 calories), you make another considerable saving.

Reducing does not mean that you must give up the foods you enjoy. You can still have the hearty meats that appeal to a masculine appetite. Just bring down their calorie counts by trimming away the fat and having them broiled or roasted instead of fried. The same principle applies to fish and poultry. A little lemon juice or a sprinkling of herbs on broiled fish or chicken gives you plenty of taste appeal without the extra calories of the butter or oil used in the frying pan. The natural juices of these foods provide a gravy you will soon learn to prefer to the thick flour and fat mixed type. Have your egg for breakfast, but remember that you add 25 to 50 calories to its basic count of 75 if you have it scrambled or fried, instead of boiled or poached.

One look at the calorie chart is all it takes to convince yourself of the calorie dangers in rich desserts. Compare any serving of pie, cake or pastry with the calorie count of a serving of fresh fruit. Say "no" to these stuffers and you will soon say "hello" to a trim, new waistline.

Reducing Diets for Men

If you are moderately active and have no glandular disturbances, you should be able to lose weight quickly, easily and safely by following a 1500 calorie plan based on the Basic Seven food groups. I suggest you divide your daily quota this way:

Breakfast:	250 calories
Lunch:	500 calories
Dinner:	600 calories
Total:	1350 calories
Bonus:	150 calories
	1500

The Bonus: The bonus is the pleasure secret of this diet plan. It provides an extra 150 calories which you may use any way you like. You might want to invest it in some crisp bacon with your morning egg, an extra serving of meat, a sample of a special sauce, an occasional glass of beer or cocktail. Choose whatever appeals to you the most. It's one way to "go off" your diet while staying on it! The bonus is enough to take the frustration out of dieting. (Incidentally, if you are inclined to be a real Spartan—and can do without spending the bonus calories—you will lose weight that much faster!)

MENU OUTLINE

BREAKFAST: 250 CALORIES

Orange juice, whole orange, ½ grapefruit or tomato juice
   or
One half cup of cereal with 1 teaspoon sugar, ¼ cup of milk
One slice whole-wheat toast or enriched bread, lightly buttered
Black coffee (saccharin sweetener if desired)

Lunch: 500 Calories

One cup vegetable, tomato, chicken or beef soup (no
creamed soup)
Mixed salad greens, 1 slice cold meat or cheese, sliced to-
matoes or
One serving lean meat, fish or poultry (not fried) and 1 serv-
ing vegetable and fresh fruit dessert
One glass skim milk or buttermilk
Black coffee or plain tea (saccharin sweetener if desired)

Dinner: 600 Calories

Tomato juice or one cup of soup (not creamed)
Or six oysters or three large shrimp
One serving lean meat, fish or poultry (not fried)
Two vegetables
Small green salad
One small piece of pie or fruit dessert
Black coffee or plain tea

Note: Eat the things you like but check the calorie counts to
make sure you are staying within your allotment. Remember
that this is only an outline and you will want to vary your
selections each day. You can trade your calories from one meal
to another occasionally but keep a close tab on the daily total.
As long as you keep to the 1500 quota, you will lose weight.

Hold That Manly Pose

Good posture is the easiest and fastest means of improving
your physical fitness and personal appearance. Back trouble is
one of the most common ailments among men. And many
backaches can be traced directly to poor posture. When you
sit and stand awkwardly, you throw an extra burden on the
sacroiliac. (Overweight adds to the pressure.) This strain, when
constant and severe, causes pressure on the sciatic nerve, bringing pain to the legs as well as the lower back.

When you slump in a chair, your weight is resting on the end of the spine instead of on the pelvic bones where it belongs. This constant pressure on the coccyx results in nerve irritation in that area and—that's right—more backaches.

Poor posture, I need hardly add, detracts from your appearance. Where is that manly chest? Caved in and hidden by slumping shoulders. Where is that tapering waist and hipline? Disguised by the sliding chest and protruding paunch.

Good posture may not turn you into an Apollo, but you will be a much more reasonable facsimile if you tighten the back muscles, throw that chest out and lift the rib cage out of the stomach. Check the difference in your mirror. Recognize that guy?

Now that you have seen what can be accomplished by diet and exercise, I hope you will be determined to begin your own program immediately — and *stick* to it. The results you achieve will be entirely up to you. While self-discipline is required at the beginning, a daily stint of exercise can become as much second nature to you as combing your hair, after a few weeks. When you see the results in your mirror, and note how much better you feel, you will never want to discontinue your program.

I hope that reading this book will mark a turning point in your life. Meanwhile, I'll see you on TV!